THE 2016 BRITISH
SUGAR FREE
SHOPPER'S GUIDE

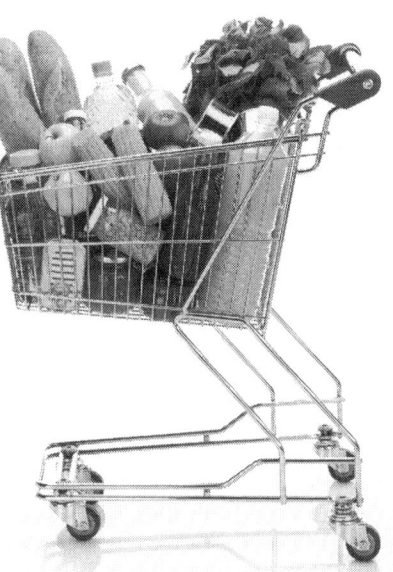

DAVID GILLESPIE

Contents

Break the Sugar Habit	2
The Important Sugars	2
A very new and deadly addition to our diet	3
How to tell if you're addicted to sugar	4
Avoiding Fructose	5
Getting Fructose Out of Your Diet	5
Sugar Substitutes	7
Seed Oils	8
The Lists	9
More Information	264

Break the Sugar Habit

Governments spend a fortune on programs aimed at making us lose weight. They tell us to eat less fatty food and exercise more. Meanwhile we fork over ever-increasing amounts on gym memberships, packaged meals, books, magazines and the advice of experts. Despite decades of this we are now fatter than at any other time in history.

Increasingly the signs are that sugar, or more specifically, fructose (the sugar in fruit, and one half of table sugar), is the culprit behind the obesity crisis.

The Important Sugars

There are only three important simple sugars: glucose, fructose and galactose. All of the other sugars you are likely to encounter in daily life are simply combinations of these three.

Glucose is by far the most plentiful of the simple sugars. Pretty much every food (except meat) contains significant quantities of glucose. Even meat (protein) is eventually converted to glucose by our digestive system. It's a pretty important sugar to humans, as it is our primary fuel – no glucose means no us.

Galactose is present in our environment in only very small quantities and is found mainly in dairy products in the form of lactose (where it is joined to a glucose molecule).

Fructose is also relatively rare in nature. It is found primarily in ripe fruits, which is why it is sometimes call fruit sugar. It is usually found together with glucose and it is what makes food taste sweet. As well as fruit, it's naturally present in honey (40%), Maple Syrup (35%) and Agave Syrup (90%).

Sucrose is what we think of when someone says table sugar. It's one half glucose and one half fructose. Brown sugar, caster sugar, raw sugar and Low GI sugar are all just sucrose.

A very new and deadly addition to our diet

Two Hundred years ago, the only way you could eat a significant amount of fructose was to be the king of England or to come into the small fortune required to buy sugar or honey. But now every person in Britain is eating just around 50 kilograms of sugar (25 kilograms of fructose) a year.

Soft-drink and fruit juice consumption alone has increased by 30 percent in just the last two decades and two thirds of the adult population is now overweight or obese. Today our collective weight problem continues to accelerate in direct proportion to our consumption of sugar.

A slew of recent research makes it clear that as a species we are ill-equipped to deal with the relatively large amounts of sugar (and therefore fructose) we now consume.

The research shows we have one primary appetite-control centre in our brain called the hypothalamus. It reacts to four major appetite hormones. Three of these hormones tell us when we have had enough to eat and one of them temporarily inhibits the effect of the other three and tells us that we need to eat.

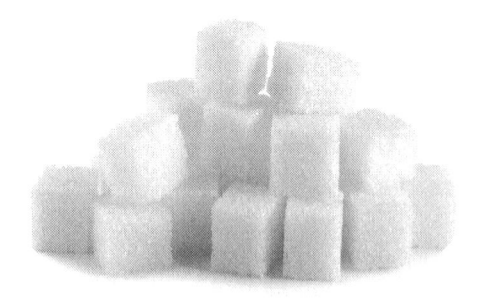

Fructose, uniquely among the food we eat, will not stimulate the release of any of the 'enough to eat' hormones. So we can eat it (and any food containing it) without feeling full. Worse still, fructose is not used for energy by our bodies. Instead all of the fructose is directly converted to fat by our livers. This means that by the time we finish our glass of apple juice (or cola or chocolate bar) the first mouthful will already be circulating in our bloodstream as fat.

Just to put the icing on the cake, recent research has now confirmed what most chocolate lovers have always suspected – sugar is as addictive as cocaine.

How to tell if you're addicted to sugar

Do you struggle to walk past a sugary treat without taking 'just one'?

Do you have routines around sugar consumption – for example, always having pudding or needing a piece of chocolate to relax in front of the TV or treating yourself to a sweet drink or chocolate after a session at the gym?

Are there are times when you feel as if you cannot go on without a sugar hit?

If you are forced to go without sugar for 24 hours, do you develop headaches and mood swings?

Obesity is just symptom of a litany of diseases caused by our fructose addiction. Some diseases are directly related to increased body weight, such as osteoarthritis, fractures, hernia and sleep apnoea. Some are related to the way in which fructose messes with our hormones, such as acne and polycystic ovary syndrome. Others are caused by the fructose induced flood of blood-borne fatty acids, notably cardiovascular diseases, fatty liver disease and type II diabetes. And recent research is also suggesting our overindulgence in fructose is directly linked to a variety of cancers, chronic kidney disease, erectile dysfunction and Alzheimer's disease.

Avoiding Fructose

The addictive ingredient in sugar is the fructose. And because it is addictive, food manufacturers have included it in just about everything.

> **Getting Fructose Out of Your Diet**
>
> Breaking a sugar addiction means that before you even start you've got to pick your way through a minefield of fructose filled foods. But in every category of foods there are some which are much lower in fructose than others. This Guide is all about helping you find those low fructose foods.

We know how difficult it is to stop smoking. Imagine how hard it would be if everything we ate or drank contained nicotine. Because much of our food is laced with fructose, breaking a sugar habit is far harder than giving up smoking. But if you use this guide to help with the shopping, you will have avoided most dietary fructose.

> **The rules for including a food are pretty simple:**
> 1. **Drinks must have no fructose per 100ml.**
> 2. **Foods must have less than 1.5g of fructose per 100g (less than 3g per 100g of 'Sugars' on the label)**

The reason for the harsh limit on drinks is that we usually drink much more than 100ml at a time. A can of soft drink is 375 ml, a bottle is 600 ml and some fast food outlets serve soft drink in 1 litre sizes. Foods on the other hand are often served at or around the hundred gram mark (except yoghurts and ice-creams which are usually 200 g).

The label on the food is the primary source for information about fructose content. "Sugars" on the label are assumed to be sucrose (glucose + fructose) unless the ingredients list indicates otherwise. For example, dairy foods will often contain considerable quantities of lactose (galactose + glucose) which will appear under the heading 'Sugars'. Those foods have the probable lactose content deducted from the sugar's total before fructose content is calculated.

If a food is not in this list then it is either too high in fructose or I am not aware of it (please send me an email david@davidgillespie.org) to let me know about any missing foods.

Only processed foods are included in the list. If you plan to eat whole food only, then you don't need to know the sugar content, just keep fruit to a minimum (less than 2 pieces per day or 1 for a child). Juice or dried versions are not acceptable substitutes for whole fruit or vegetables.

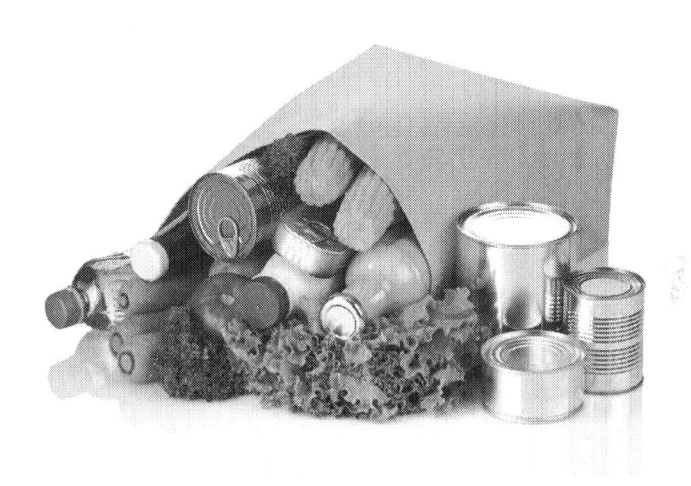

Sugar Substitutes

I'm not a big fan of the term artificial sweetener. It implies that other sweeteners (such as sugar, or fruit juice or high fructose corn syrup) are in some way natural, with all the goodness we have been conditioned to imply into that term. And there is nothing natural about extracting sugar from sugar cane. Substitute sweetener strikes me as a more appropriate description. They are substitutes for sugar, intended to do the job of sugar. In reality sugar itself is a substitute sweetener (for honey) but let's not get all technical. They are all created by using various levels of technology (from manmade beehives to industrial chemical plants) with the sole purpose of adding sweet taste to foods which are not otherwise sweet.

There are three categories of substitute sweetener; those that are absolutely safe to consume; and those that may be safe in limited doses and those which are not safe under any circumstances (usually because they are metabolized to fructose anyway).

Substitute Sweeteners commonly used in Britain

Good	Your call	Bad	
Corn Syrup	Acesulphame potassium (#950)	Agave Syrup	Mannitol (#421)
Dextrose	Alitame (#956)	Fructose	Maple Syrup
Glucose	Aspartame (#951)	Fruit Juice Extract	Molasses
Glucose Syrup	Aspartame-acesuphame (#962)	Golden Syrup	Polydextrose
Lactose	Cyclamates (#952)	High Fructose Corn Syrup	Resistant (malto) dextrin
Maltose	Erythritol (#968)	Honey	Sorbitol (#420)
Maltodextrin	Neotame (#961)	Inulin	Sucrose
Maltodextrose	Saccharin (#954)	Isomalt (#953)	Wheat dextrin
Rice Malt Syrup	Stevia (#960)	Lactitol (#966)	
	Sucralose (#955)	Litesse	
	Xylitol (#967)	Maltitol (#965)	

Seed Oils

The lists that follow are based entirely on sugar content alone. I have also written about the dangers of some types of vegetable oil (seed oils) in my book *Toxic Oil*. Some of the products in the lists below will contain seed oils, but as food manufacturers are not required to label the exact fats that they are using in a product, I have not included information about the fats in these lists. We can however have an educated guess and if you are concerned about the seed oil content of any product, I encourage you to use my fat ready reckoner chart available at www.howmuchsugar.com.

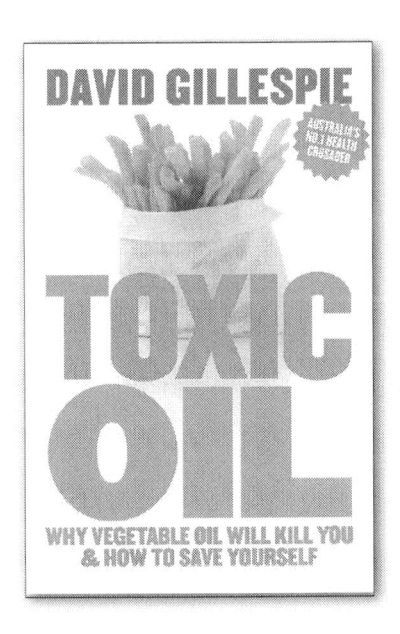

The Lists

Cereal Bars	11
Drinks	11
Confectionery	12
Condiments	13
Cooking Sauces	18
Breakfast Cereals	
Breakfast Cereals – by sugar content	26
Breakfast Cereals – by brand	31
Ice-Cream	36
Yoghurts	
Yoghurts – by sugar content	37
Yoghurts – by brand	45
Breads	
Breads – by sugar content	53
Breads – by brand	53

Biscuits

Biscuits – by sugar content	81
Biscuits – by brand	94

Frozen Pizza

Frozen Pizza – by sugar content	107
Frozen Pizza – by brand	114

Ready Meals

Ready Meals – by sugar content	120
Ready Meals – by brand	182

Fast Food

Subway Restaurants	239
McDonald's	243
Burger King	245
Pizza Hut	246
Domino's Pizza	255
KFC	256
Pret a Manger	257
EAT	260

Cereal Bars

No qualifying products.

The Atkins Advantage brand of bars are very low in sugar but use artificial sweeteners which are metabolized to fructose (the one's on the 'your call' list on previous page).

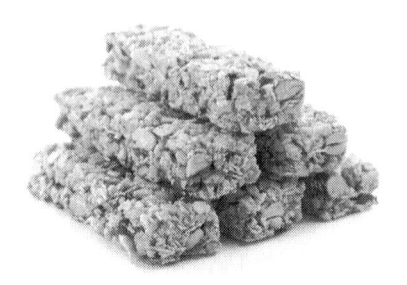

Drinks

The only qualifying products are unsweetened tea or coffee, diet soft drinks, water and milk (both whole and low fat).

The only branded soft drink which qualifies as low fructose is Lucozade Original. It is sweetened with glucose (only) and therefore contains no fructose.

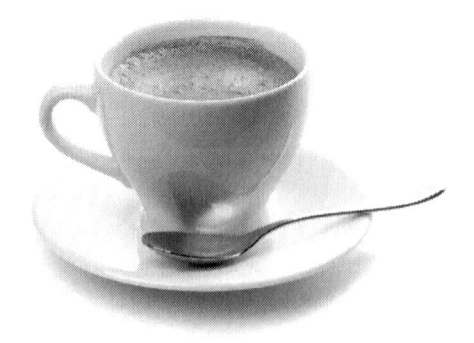

Confectionery

All of the following products have been sweetened with glucose rather than sugar (sucrose).

Maker	Product
Wonka (Nestle)	Runts
	Bottle Caps
	Everlasting Gobstopper
	Chewy Gobstopper
	Gobstopper Snowballs
Frusano	Filita Organic Whole Milk Chocolate
	Organic-Filita Amaranth
	Organic Rice-Crispies
	Filita Organic Dark Chocolate
	Organic Fili-Bears (Gummi Bears)
	Organic Blackberry Candies
	Organic Peppermint Candies
	Ricemalt peppermint hard candy
	Ricemalt lemon hard candy
	Ricemalt orange hard candy
	Dextrose Lolly

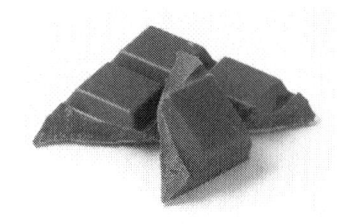

Condiments

These have been arranged by type and then by brand. You'll see that there are no options for some of the more common table sauces like Ketchup and BBQ Sauce. If you want those you'll have to make them yourself. I have provided some easy-to-make recipes in *The Sweet Poison Quit Plan*. It is safest to assume that all of these products contain seed oils except the Mustards.

Brand	Label	% Sugar
	MAYONNAISE	
ASDA	Chosen by you Mayonnaise	1.8 %
	Chosen by you Mustard Mayo	2.6 %
Atkins & Potts	Classic Mayonnaise	1.7 %
	Fiery Wasabi Mayonnaise	2.0 %
	Smoky & Spicy Chipotle Chilli Mayonnaise	2.0 %
	Yummy Toasted Garlic Mayonnaise	1.7 %
	Zesty Lemon Mayonnaise	1.8 %
Biona Organic	Sunflower Oil Mayonnaise	1.5 %
	Wasabi Style Mayonnaise	1.5 %
Delouis	Garlic Mayonnaise	0.3 %
	Mayonnaise	0.3 %
Gefen	Lite Mayonnaise	0.0 %
Gran Luchito	Smoked Chilli Mayo	0.2 %
Heinz	Magnificent Mayonnaise	2.9 %
Hellmann's	Light Mayonnaise	2.3 %
	Mayonnaise with a Pinch of Mustard	2.5 %
	Mayonnaise with a Touch of Garlic	2.2 %
	Mayonnaise with a Zing of Lemon	2.3 %
	Real Mayonnaise	1.3 %

Brand	Label	% Sugar
Hillfarm	Garlic Mayonnaise	3.0 %
Maille	Mayonnaise with a Hint of Mustard	1.0 %
Mellow Yellow	Mayonnaise	2.8 %
Morrisons	Garlic Mayo	1.2 %
	Light Mayonnaise	2.7 %
	Mayonnaise	1.4 %
	Savers Mayonnaise	2.2 %
Sainsbury's	Be Good Mayonnaise	2.9 %
	French Style Mayonnaise	2.0 %
	Light Mayonnaise	2.7 %
	Mayonnaise	1.0 %
	SO Organic Mayonnaise	2.3 %
	Taste the Difference Mayonnaise	2.5 %
Saitaku	Wasabi Mayonnaise	2.0 %
Simply Delicious	Organic Garlic Mayonnaise	2.0 %
Stokes	Blushed Tomato Mayonnaise	2.2 %
	Chilli Mayonnaise	1.7 %
	Garlic Mayonnaise	2.0 %
	Herb Mayonnaise	1.6 %
	Lemon Mayonnaise	1.8 %
	Real Mayonnaise	1.6 %
Tesco	Finest Mayonnaise with Extra Virgin Olive Oil	2.4 %
	Finest Roasted Garlic & Cracked Black Pepper Mayonnaise	2.7 %
	French Style Mayonnaise	1.5 %
	Light Mayonnaise	2.5 %
	Mayonnaise	1.4 %

Brand	Label	% Sugar
Tesco	Organic Mayonnaise	1.8 %
The Bay Tree	Classic Mayonnaise	0.0 %
Tracklements	Mayonnaise	0.0 %
Waitrose	Essential Mayonnaise	2.3 %
	Mayonnaise with Extra Virgin Olive Oil	1.8 %
	Organic Mayonnaise	2.1 %
Winiary	Majonez	2.6 %

MUSTARDS

Brand	Label	% Sugar
ASDA	Extra Special Tewkesbury Mustard	2.5 %
Atkins & Potts	Classic Dijon Mustard	0.0 %
	Essential Wholegrain Mustard	0.0 %
Beaver Brand	American Picnic Mustard	2.8 %
Biona Organic	Horseradish Mustard	2.6 %
Bornier	Dijon Mustard	2.7 %
French's	Classic Yellow Mustard	1.0 %
	Smooth & Spicy American Mustard	1.3 %
Heinz	Smooth & Mild Mustard	3.0 %
Maille	Mustard with Horseradish	1.0 %
	Traditional Dijon Mustard	1.9 %
Morrisons	Dijon Mustard	2.1 %
Sainsbury's	Dijon Mustard	2.5 %
	French Mustard	2.8 %
	Horseradish Mustard	2.7 %
Tesco	Dijon Mustard	1.0 %
	Finest Dijon Mustard with White Wine	2.3 %
	Finest Wholegrain Mustard with White Wine	2.2 %
	Wholegrain Mustard	2.7 %

Brand	Label	% Sugar
The East India Company	Bulldog Mustard	0.2 %
	Lapsang Souchong Mustard	1.2 %
The East India Company	Mrs Clements English Mustard	0.1 %
The English Provender Co.	Wholegrain Mustard with Horseradish	1.8 %
Tracklements	Dijon Mustard	1.8 %
Waitrose	Duchy Original Organic Wholegrain Mustard with Honey	2.6 %
	Essential Dijon Mustard	2.7 %
	Essential English Mustard	2.9 %
	Essential Wholegrain Mustard	2.3 %
DRESSINGS		
Atkins & Potts	Classic Herb & Garlic Dressing	2.3 %
Cardini's	Caesar Dressing	0.3 %
	Light Caesar Dressing	2.0 %
	Ranch Dressing	2.3 %
Hellmann's	Caesar Dressing	2.2 %
Newman's Own	Caesar Dressing	0.6 %
	Italian Dressing	0.3 %
Pizza Express	House Dressing	2.7 %
Righteous	Mild English Blue Cheese & Cider Dressing	2.6 %
Sainsbury's	Be Good Blue Cheese Dressing	2.9 %
Tesco	Caesar Dressing	2.7 %
Waitrose	Half Fat Olive Oil Dressing	3.0 %
OTHERS		
Cholula	Chili Garlic Hot Sauce	0.0 %
	Chili Lime Hot Sauce	0.0 %

Brand	Label	% Sugar
Cholula	Chipotle Hot Sauce	0.0 %
	Green Pepper Hot Sauce	0.0 %
	Original Hot Sauce	0.0 %
Frank's	Red Hot Chilli 'N Lime Sauce	0.7 %
	Red Hot Wings Buffalo Sauce	0.6 %
	Red Hot Wings Hot Buffalo Sauce	0.0 %
Heinz	Lively & Fruity Hot Pepper Sauce	3.0 %
Levi Roots	Scotch Bonnet Chilli Sauce	1.2 %
Morrisons	Takeaway Garlic Sauce	1.8 %
Newman's Own	Hot Pepper Sauce	0.7 %
Sainsbury's	Hollandaise Sauce	3.0 %
	Peri Peri Sauce	2.7 %

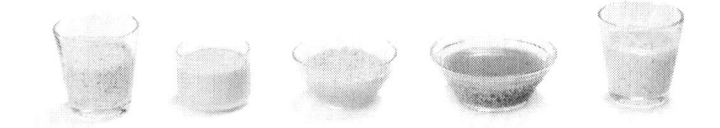

Cooking Sauces

These sauces are arranged by cooking style and then by brand and then by sugar content. Many of them contain seed oils. So be careful if you are also aiming to avoid them.

Brand	Label	% Sugar
	ASIAN	
ASDA	Curry Sauce Instant Sauce Mix	2.0 %
	Curry Sauce Mix	2.2 %
	Green Thai Style Cooking Sauce	2.9 %
	Red Thai Cooking Sauce	2.6 %
Morrisons	Chinese Curry Cooking Sauce	2.9 %
Sainsbury's	Basics Chicken Curry	2.8 %
	Butter Chicken Cooking Sauce	3.0 %
Sharwood's	Chinese Curry Cooking Sauce	2.9 %
Thai Taste	Chilli & Holy Basil Stir Fry Sauce	1.7 %
	Easy Thai Green Curry Kit	0.7 %
	Easy Thai Red Curry Kit	0.7 %
	Gang Keow Wan Green Curry Sauce	2.8 %
	Penang Red Curry Sauce	2.7 %
Tiger Tiger	Thai Green Curry Simmer Sauce	1.9 %
	Thai Red Curry Simmer Sauce	2.8 %
	ITALIAN	
ASDA	Green Pesto Sauce	2.2 %
	Lasagne Topper	2.2 %
	Reduced Fat Green Pesto Sauce	0.4 %
	Smartprice Bolognese Sauce	1.7 %
Biona Organic	Green Pesto with Pine Kernels	0.9 %

Brand	Label	% Sugar
David & Oliver	Venison, Mushroom & Whisky Pasta Sauce	0.9 %
	Wild Boar Ragu Pasta Sauce	2.3 %
Dolmio	Express Creamy Carbonara Pasta Sauce	1.2 %
	Express Creamy Mushroom Pasta Sauce	1.4 %
	Lasagne Cheesy Sauce	2.2 %
	Lasagne Creamy Sauce	2.6 %
	Macaroni Cheese Pasta Bake	2.1 %
	Stir-in Creamy Carbonara Pasta Sauce	1.1 %
Homepride	Cheesy Pasta Bake Sauce	1.6 %
Jamie Oliver	Chilli & Garlic Pesto	2.9 %
	Coriander & Cashew Pesto	1.9 %
	Green Pesto	2.6 %
	Italian Herb Pesto	1.7 %
Loyd Grossman	Creamy White Lasagne Sauce	0.8 %
Meena	Risotto al Funghi with Porcini Mushrooms Sauce	2.9 %
Morrisons	Carbonara Pasta Sauce	0.0 %
	M Kitchen Italian Bolognese	2.4 %
	M Kitchen Italian Carbonara	1.4 %
	M Kitchen Italian Cheese Sauce	2.8 %
	M Kitchen Italian Creamy Mushroom	0.7 %
	M Kitchen Italian Tomato & Mascarpone	2.7 %
	Savers Pasta Sauce	0.9 %
	Signature Creamy Four Cheese	2.2 %
	Signature Creamy Tomato & Mascarpone	2.5 %
	Spinach & Ricotta Pasta Sauce	0.7 %
	White Lasagne Sauce	0.4 %
	White Wine Sauce	1.8 %

Brand	Label	% Sugar
Ragu	White Lasagne Sauce	2 %
Sacla Italia	Al Forno Four Italian Cheese & Black Summer Truffle Bake Sauce	1.9 %
	Al Forno Italian Tomato, Roasted Pepper & Fiery Red Chilli Bake Sauce	2.1 %
	Free From Tomato Pesto	1.7 %
	Fresh Coriander Pesto	0.8 %
	Intenso Tomato & Olive Stir In Sauce	2.7 %
	Kale & Smoked Ricotta Pesto	2.0 %
	Organic Basil Pesto	1.4 %
	Roasted Pepper Pesto	2.3 %
	Wild Garlic Pesto	1.9 %
	Wild Rocket Pesto	2.3 %
Sainsbury's	Basics Pasta Sauce	1.8 %
	Carbonara Pasta Sauce	0.5 %
	Cheesy White Lasagne Sauce	0.5 %
	Creamy Leak & Bacon Pasta Bake Sauce	1.7 %
	Creamy Mushroom Pasta Bake Sauce	1.7 %
	Creamy White Lasagne Sauce	0.5 %
	Four Cheese Pasta Sauce	0.5 %
	Green Pesto	1.0 %
	Italian Carbonara Sauce	1.2 %
	Italian Green Pesto	0.5 %
	Italian Mushroom Sauce	1.8 %
	Italian Spinach & Ricotta Sauce	1.7 %
	Italian Three Cheese Sauce	2.0 %
	Macaroni Cheese Pasta Bake Sauce	2.1 %
	Spinach & Ricotta Pesto	2.4 %
	Taste the Difference Carbonara Sauce	2.1 %

Brand	Label	% Sugar
Sainsbury's	Taste the Difference Pesto Alla Genovese	0.5 %
Santa Maria	Mexican Meatballs Sauce	3.0 %
Schwartz	Lasagne Recipe Mix	1.2 %
Tesco	Carbonara Pasta Sauce	0.1 %
	Classic Green Pesto	2.6 %
	Everyday Value Pasta Sauce	2.3 %
	Finest Pesto Alla Genovese	2.2 %
	Reduced Fat Green Pesto	0.4 %
	White Lasagne Pasta Sauce	0.1 %
Tideford	Organic Basil Pesto	0.5 %
	Organic Carbonara Sauce with Bacon & Nutmeg	2.2 %
	Organic Ragu A La Bolognese	2.7 %
Waitrose	A Romantic Green Pesto with Basil	0.4 %
	Bright & Green Basil Pesto	0.5 %
	Creamy Asparagus Pasta Sauce	2.2 %
	Creamy Carbonara Sauce with Pancetta	1.7 %
	Creamy Mushroom Sauce with Porcini	0.7 %
	Flavoursome Pesto alla Genovese	0.4 %
	Intense & Silky Carbonara Sauce	2.5 %
	Intense Puttanesca Sauce with Olives & Anchovies	2.9 %
	Menu Intense Green Pesto	0.7 %
	Rich Beef Bolognese Sauce with Tomato	2.7 %
	White Lasagne Sauce	0.6 %
Weight Watchers	Tomato And Basil Sauce	3.0 %
	INDIAN	
ASDA	Balti Cooking Sauce	2.5 %
	Fruity Biryani Oven Bake Sauce	2.1 %

Brand	Label	% Sugar
ASDA	Madras Cooking Sauce	1.0 %
Loyd Grossman	Bhuna Cooking Sauce	2.8 %
	Madras Cooking Sauce	2.7 %
Our Little Secret	Exquisite Kashmiri Roganjosh Cooking Sauce	1.0 %
	Indian Bengal Shorshe Jhol Cooking Sauce	1.7 %
	Tantalising Punjab Jalfrezi Cooking Sauce	2.6 %
	Temptuous Tikka Labadar Cooking Sauce	0.9 %
Patak's	Spice Sensation's Vibrant Vindaloo Cooking Sauce	
Sharwood's	Extra Onions Tikka Masala	1.1 %
	Lime Pickle Cooking Sauce	1.6 %
	Vindaloo Cooking Sauce	2.6 %
Tesco	Healthy Living Rogan Josh Cooking Sauce	2.5 %
	Saag Aloo Sauce	2.6 %
The Hairy Dieters	Our Cooking Sauce Chicken Korma	2.7 %
	Our Cooking Sauce Lamb Saag Curry	2.7 %
The Spice Tailor	Keralan Coconut Curry	3.0 %
	Mangalore Herb Curry	2.9 %
	Spiced Spinach Curry	1.9 %
TRADITIONAL		
ASDA	Beef & Ale Slow Cook Sauce	1.6 %
	Carbonara Pasta Sauce	1.1 %
	Cheese & Bacon Pasta Bake Sauce	1.5 %
	Cheese Sauce Mix	1.0 %
	Creamy Garlic Pour Over Sauce	2.5 %
	Creamy Mushroom Pour Over Sauce	1.6 %
	Dauphinoise Potato Bake Cooking Sauce	2.9 %

Brand	Label	% Sugar
ASDA	Gluten Free Cheese Simmer Sauce Mix	3.0 %
	Gluten Free Parsley Simmer Sauce Mix	2.5 %
	Gluten Free White Simmer Sauce Mix	2.5 %
	Instant Cheese Sauce Mix	1.3 %
	Instant Onion & Chive Sauce Mix	0.9 %
	Instant Parsley Sauce Mix	1.2 %
	Macaroni Cheese Pasta Bake	1.5 %
	Peppercorn Pour Over Sauce	1.6 %
	Peppercorn Sauce Mix	0.3 %
	Stroganoff Cooking Sauce	2.6 %
	White Wine & Cream Cooking Sauce	1.8 %
Atkins & Potts	Wild Mushroom & Tarragon Pasta Sauce	2.1 %
Chicken Tonight	Chasseur One Pan Sauce	3.0 %
	Country French One Pan Sauce	2.3 %
	Creamy Mushroom One Pan Sauce	1.7 %
Homepride	Chasseur Cooking Sauce	2.6 %
	Cheese & Ham Potato Bake Sauce	1.0 %
	Chicken Casserole Cook-In Sauce	2.7 %
	Chicken Chasseur Cooking Sauce	2.7 %
	Chicken Supreme Cook-In-Sauce	1.5 %
	Classic Recipe White Wine & Cream Cooking Sauce	2.4 %
	Creamy Carbonara Pasta Bake Sauce	0.9 %
	Creamy Mushroom Sauce	1.5 %
	Creamy Peppercorn Cook-In-Sauce	2.2 %
	Creamy White Wine Sauce	1.6 %
	Garlic & Herb Potato Bake Sauce	0.8 %
	Lemon & Herb Cooking Sauce	2.2 %

Brand	Label	% Sugar
Loyd Grossman	Carbonara Express Sauce	0.9 %
	Classics Bourguignon Cooking Sauce	1.0 %
	Classics Coq Au Vin Cooking Sauce	1.1 %
	Creamy Mushroom Express Sauce	0.5 %
	Creamy Parmesan & Cheddar Pour Over Sauce	0.9 %
	Creamy Peppercorn & Brandy Pour Over Sauce	1.7 %
	Gastro Beef & Ale Cooking Sauce	2.3 %
	Gastro Creamy Leek & Bacon Cooking Sauce	1.5 %
	White Wine & Parsley Pour Over Sauce	1.4 %
	Wholegrain Mustard & Tarragon Pour Over Sauce	1.8 %
Morrisons	Beef in Ale Sauce	2.1 %
	Diane Sauce	1.5 %
	Peppercorn Sauce	2.8 %
Ragu	Cheese & Bacon Pasta Bake Sauce	2.1 %
Raymond Blanc	Mustard Pour Over Sauce	1.0 %
	Peppercorn Pour Over Sauce	2.6 %
Sainsbury's	Beef & Ale Cooking Sauce	1.8 %
	Creamy Cheese & Bacon Potato Bake Sauce	1.7 %
	Creamy Mushroom Cooking Sauce	1.6 %
	Creamy White Wine Cooking Sauce	2.9 %
Schwartz	Cheddar Cheese Sauce Mix	1.3 %
	Chicken & Leek Bake Recipe Mix	2.1 %
	Chicken Casserole Recipe Mix	1.2 %
	Chicken Chasseur Recipe Mix	1.5 %
	Creamy Mild Peppercorn Sauce Mix	2.1 %

Brand	Label	% Sugar
Schwartz	Creamy Parsley Sauce Mix	1.5 %
	Creamy Pepper Sauce Mix	1.7 %
	Dauphinoise Potato Bake Recipe Mix	0.7 %
	Garlic, Mushroom & Cream Sauce Mix	1.2 %
	Heat & Pour Creamy Pepper Sauce	0.9 %
	Heat & Pour Mushroom Sauce	1.1 %
	Hollandaise Sauce Mix	0.8 %
	Savoury Mince Recipe Mix	2.4 %
	Spaghetti Carbonara Recipe Mix	2.0 %
	Winter Recipe Creamy Cheese & Ham Pasta Bake Sauce Mix	0.6 %
Tesco	Cider & Mustard Pour Over Sauce	2.9 %
	Diane Pour Over Sauce	2.0 %
Tideford	Organic Westcountry Cheese Sauce	2.0 %
Waitrose	Cooks' Ingredients Bechamel Sauce	2.3 %
	Essential Cheese Sauce	1.0 %
	Rich Four Cheese Sauce	2.2 %
	Tomato & Mascarpone with Wensleydale Cheese Favourite Sauces	2.7 %

MEXICAN/SPANISH

Brand	Label	% Sugar
ASDA	Mexican Style Cowboy Chilli Cooking Sauce	2.5 %
Santa Maria	Enchilada Sauce	3.0 %
Schwartz	Hot Chilli con Carne Recipe Mix	2.7 %
Tesco	Everyday Value Chilli Con Carne Sauce	2.5 %
Weight Watchers	Chilli Con Carne Cooking Sauce	2.7 %
	Spanish Chicken Cooking Sauce	2.7

Breakfast Cereals

I've presented this list in two formats so you can browse by sugar content or brand.

Breakfast Cereals - by sugar content

Brand	Label	% Sugar
Rude Health	Sprouted Porridge Oats	0.0 %
Delicious Alchemy	Rice Flake Porridge	0.1 %
Rude Health	Spelt Flakes Cereal	0.5 %
Rude Health	Puffed Oats Cereal	0.6 %
Sainsbury's	Puffed Wheat	0.6 %
Sainsbury's	Wholegrain Mini Wheats	0.6 %
White's	Toat'ly Oaty Original Jumbo Porridge Oats	0.6 %
Doves Farm	Corn Flakes	0.7 %
Kallo	Wholegrain Breakfast Puffs	0.7 %
Nature's Store	Puffed Rice Cereal	0.7 %
Nestle	Shredded Wheat Bitesize	0.7 %
Nestle	Shredded Wheat Original	0.7 %
Rude Health	5 Grain 5 Seed Porridge	0.7 %
Rude Health	Puffed Brown Rice Cereal	0.7 %
White's	Organic Traditional Oats	0.7 %
Rude Health	Daily Oats Porridge	0.9 %
Sainsbury's	Oatbran & Wheatbran Scottish Porridge Oats	0.9 %
Tesco	Original Easy Oats	0.9 %
Amisa Organic	Gluten Free Pure Porridge Oats	1.0 %
ASDA	Ready Oats	1.0 %

Breakfast Cereals - by sugar content (continued)

Brand	Label	% Sugar
Flahavan's	Jumbo Oat Flakes	1.0 %
Flahavan's	Natural Quick Oats	1.0 %
Flahavan's	Organic Jumbo Oats	1.0 %
Flahavan's	Organic Porridge Oats	1.0 %
Flahavan's	Organic Quick Oats	1.0 %
Flahavan's	Pinhead Oatmeal	1.0 %
Flahavan's	Progress Oatlets	1.0 %
Jordans	Chunky Traditional Organic Porridge	1.0 %
Jordans	Chunky Traditional Porridge	1.0 %
Jordans	Quick & Creamy Porridge	1.0 %
M (Morrisons)	M Savers Porridge Oats	1.0 %
M (Morrisons)	Original Oats	1.0 %
M (Morrisons)	Porridge Oats	1.0 %
Mornflake	Coarse Oatmeal	1.0 %
Mornflake	Jumbo Oats	1.0 %
Mornflake	Oats 2 Go Original Porridge	1.0 %
Mornflake	Organic Oats	1.0 %
Mornflake	Scottish Jumbo Oats	1.0 %
Mornflake	Stoneground Fine Oatmeal	1.0 %
Mornflake	Stoneground Medium Oatmeal	1.0 %
Mornflake	Superfast Oats	1.0 %
Quaker	Oat So Simple Original Porridge	1.0 %
Rude Health	The Oatmeal Porridge	1.0 %
Sainsbury's	Original Express Porridge	1.0 %
Sainsbury's	Ready Oats	1.0 %
Sainsbury's	SO Organic Original Express Porridge	1.0 %

Breakfast Cereals - by sugar content (continued)

Brand	Label	% Sugar
Sainsbury's	SO Organic Porridge Oats	1.0 %
Scott's	Original Porage Oats	1.0 %
Scott's	So-Easy Original Porage Oats	1.0 %
Stoats	Apple & Cinnamon Porridge	1.0 %
Stoats	Scottish Porridge	1.0 %
Tesco	Chunky Oats & Barley Easy Oats	1.0 %
Tesco	Instant Hot Oat Cereal	1.0 %
Tesco	Organic Porridge Oats	1.0 %
The Food Doctor	Multigrain & Seed Porridge	1.0 %
Waitrose	Organic Rolled Jumbo Oats	1.0 %
Weetabix	Ready Brek Original Porridge	1.0 %
White's	Extra Fine Oat Bran	1.0 %
White's	Medium Cut Oat Bran	1.0 %
Quaker	100 % Wholegrain Rolled Oats	1.1 %
Quaker	Jumbo Whole Rolled Oats	1.1 %
Sainsbury's	Scottish Porridge Oats	1.1 %
Sainsbury's	Taste the Difference Whole Rolled Porridge Oats	1.1 %
Scott's	Old Fashioned Porage Oats	1.1 %
Tesco	Finest Scottish Porridge Oats	1.1 %
Tesco	Scottish Porridge Oats	1.1 %
Waitrose	Essential Original Instant Oats	1.1 %
Amisa Organic	Gluten Free Four Grain Porridge	1.2 %
ASDA	Free From Pure Porridge Oats	1.2 %
ASDA	Simply Scottish Original Porridge	1.2 %
ASDA	Simply Scottish Wholemeal Porridge	1.2 %

Breakfast Cereals – by sugar content (continued)

Brand	Label	% Sugar
Fuel	Protibrick Wheat Biscuits	1.2 %
Mornflake	Gluten Free Jumbo Oats	1.2 %
Mornflake	Gluten Free Pinhead Oatmeal	1.2 %
Mornflake	Gluten Free Porridge Oats	1.2 %
Mornflake	Oatbran	1.2 %
Mornflake	Oatbran Sprinkles	1.2 %
Flahavan's	Multiseed Porridge	1.3 %
Flahavan's	Multiseed Quick Oats	1.3 %
Flahavan's	Oat Bran	1.3 %
ASDA	Smart Price Porridge Oats	1.3 %
Ella's Kitchen	Wakey Wakey Round Ones Cereal	1.3 %
M (Morrisons)	Puffed Wheat	1.3 %
Tesco	Oatbran	1.3 %
White's	Organic Jumbo Oats	1.4 %
Amisa Organic	Gluten Free Quinoa Flakes Cereal	1.5 %
Biona Organic	Amaranth Pops Cereal	1.5 %
Mornflake	Toasted Oatbran	1.5 %
Tesco	Everyday Value Porridge Oats	1.5 %
Waitrose	Essential Porridge Oats	1.5 %
Waitrose	Love Life Muesli Base	1.5 %
Waitrose	Scottish Porridge Oats with Bran	1.5 %
White's	Speedicook Porridge Oats	1.6 %
Stoats	Sunflower & Poppy Seed Porridge	1.7 %
Waitrose	Duchy Originals Organic Oat & Barley Porridge	1.7 %
Sainsbury's	Chunky Oats & Barley Express Porridge	1.8 %

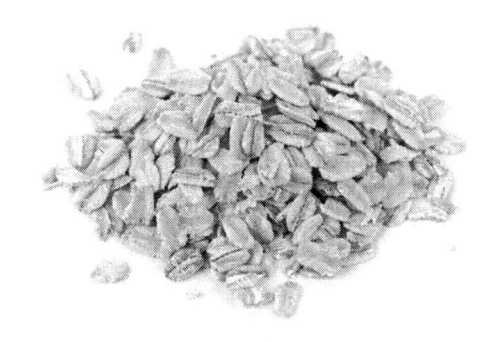

Breakfast Cereals - by sugar content (continued)

Brand	Label	% Sugar
The Good Grain Co.	Puffed Wheat	2.0 %
Sainsbury's	SO Organic Cornflakes	2.1 %
ASDA	Kids Scrummy Porridge Sachets	2.2 %
Amisa Organic	Spelt Puffs Cereal	2.3 %
Jordans	Natural Wheat Bran	2.3 %
Jordans	Natural Wheat Bran	2.3 %
ASDA	Smart Price Wheat Bisks	2.5 %
M (Morrisons)	M Savers Wheat Biscuits	2.5 %
Sainsbury's	Basics Breakfast Wholewheat Biscuits	2.5 %

Breakfast Cereals – by brand

Brand	Label	% Sugar
Amisa Organic	Gluten Free Four Grain Porridge	1.2 %
	Gluten Free Pure Porridge Oats	1.0 %
	Gluten Free Quinoa Flakes Cereal	1.5 %
	Spelt Puffs Cereal	2.3 %
ASDA	Free From Pure Porridge Oats	1.2 %
	Kids Scrummy Porridge Sachets	2.2 %
	Ready Oats	1.0 %
	Simply Scottish Original Porridge	1.2 %
	Simply Scottish Wholemeal Porridge	1.2 %
	Smart Price Porridge Oats	1.3 %
	Smart Price Wheat Bisks	2.5 %
Biona Organic	Amaranth Pops Cereal	1.5 %
Delicious Alchemy	Rice Flake Porridge	0.1 %
Doves Farm	Corn Flakes	0.7 %
Ella's Kitchen	Wakey Wakey Round Ones Cereal	1.3 %
Flahavan's	Jumbo Oat Flakes	1.0 %
	Multiseed Porridge	1.3 %
	Multiseed Quick Oats	1.3 %
	Natural Quick Oats	1.0 %
	Oat Bran	1.3 %
	Organic Jumbo Oats	1.0 %
	Organic Porridge Oats	1.0 %
	Organic Quick Oats	1.0 %
	Pinhead Oatmeal	1.0 %
	Progress Oatlets	1.0 %

Breakfast Cereals – by brand (continued)

Brand	Label	% Sugar
Fuel	Protibrick Wheat Biscuits	1.2 %
Jordans	Chunky Traditional Organic Porridge	1.0 %
	Chunky Traditional Porridge	1.0 %
	Natural Wheat Bran	2.3 %
	Natural Wheat Bran	2.3 %
	Quick & Creamy Porridge	1.0 %
Kallo	Wholegrain Breakfast Puffs	0.7 %
M (Morrisons)	M Savers Porridge Oats	1.0 %
	M Savers Wheat Biscuits	2.5 %
	Original Oats	1.0 %
	Porridge Oats	1.0 %
	Puffed Wheat	1.3 %
Mornflake	Coarse Oatmeal	1.0 %
	Gluten Free Jumbo Oats	1.2 %
	Gluten Free Pinhead Oatmeal	1.2 %
	Gluten Free Porridge Oats	1.2 %
	Jumbo Oats	1.0 %
	Oatbran	1.2 %
	Oatbran Sprinkles	1.2 %
	Oats 2 Go Original Porridge	1.0 %
	Organic Oats	1.0 %
	Scottish Jumbo Oats	1.0 %
	Stoneground Fine Oatmeal	1.0 %
	Stoneground Medium Oatmeal	1.0 %
	Superfast Oats	1.0 %
	Toasted Oatbran	1.5 %

Breakfast Cereals - by brand (continued)

Brand	Label	% Sugar
Nature's Store	Puffed Rice Cereal	0.7 %
Nestle	Shredded Wheat Bitesize	0.7 %
	Shredded Wheat Original	0.7 %
Quaker	100 % Wholegrain Rolled Oats	1.1 %
	Jumbo Whole Rolled Oats	1.1 %
	Oat So Simple Original Porridge	1.0 %
Rude Health	5 Grain 5 Seed Porridge	0.7 %
	Daily Oats Porridge	0.9 %
	Puffed Brown Rice Cereal	0.7 %
	Puffed Oats Cereal	0.6 %
	Spelt Flakes Cereal	0.5 %
	Sprouted Porridge Oats	0.0 %
	The Oatmeal Porridge	1.0 %
Sainsbury's	Basics Breakfast Wholewheat Biscuits	2.5 %
	Chunky Oats & Barley Express Porridge	1.8 %
	Oatbran & Wheatbran Scottish Porridge Oats	0.9 %
	Original Express Porridge	1.0 %
	Puffed Wheat	0.6 %
	Ready Oats	1.0 %
	Scottish Porridge Oats	1.1 %
	SO Organic Cornflakes	2.1 %
	SO Organic Original Express Porridge	1.0 %
	SO Organic Porridge Oats	1.0 %
	Taste the Difference Whole Rolled Porridge Oats	1.1 %
	Wholegrain Mini Wheats	0.6 %

Breakfast Cereals – by brand (continued)

Brand	Label	% Sugar
Scott's	Old Fashioned Porage Oats	1.1 %
	Original Porage Oats	1.0 %
	So-Easy Original Porage Oats	1.0 %
Stoats	Apple & Cinnamon Porridge	1.0 %
	Scottish Porridge	1.0 %
	Sunflower & Poppy Seed Porridge	1.7 %
Tesco	Chunky Oats & Barley Easy Oats	1.0 %
	Everyday Value Porridge Oats	1.5 %
	Finest Scottish Porridge Oats	1.1 %
	Instant Hot Oat Cereal	1.0 %
	Oatbran	1.3 %
	Organic Porridge Oats	1.0 %
	Original Easy Oats	0.9 %
	Scottish Porridge Oats	1.1 %
The Food Doctor	Multigrain & Seed Porridge	1.0 %
The Good Grain Co.	Puffed Wheat	2.0 %
Waitrose	Duchy Originals Organic Oat & Barley Porridge	1.7 %
	Essential Original Instant Oats	1.1 %
	Essential Porridge Oats	1.5 %
	Love Life Muesli Base	1.5 %
	Organic Rolled Jumbo Oats	1.0 %
	Scottish Porridge Oats with Bran	1.5 %
Weetabix	Ready Brek Original Porridge	1.0 %
White's	Extra Fine Oat Bran	1.0 %

Breakfast Cereals – by brand (continued)

Brand	Label	% Sugar
White's	Medium Cut Oat Bran	1.0 %
	Organic Jumbo Oats	1.4 %
	Organic Traditional Oats	0.7 %
	Speedicook Porridge Oats	1.6 %
	Toat'ly Oaty Original Jumbo Porridge Oats	0.6 %

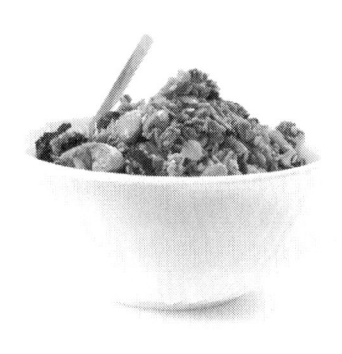

Ice-Cream

You won't be surprised to find that there no store bought ice-creams which satisfy the rule. Even a small bowl (200 g) of the lowest-sugar ice-cream (Weight Watchers Toffee & Honeycomb Sundae) delivers four teaspoons of added sugar. You'll be pleased to discover that I do provide a great recipe for sugar-free ice-cream in the recipe sections of www.howmuchsugar.com, in the *Quit Plan Cookbook* and in the *Sweet Poison Quit Plan*. Unfortunately, however, you have to make it yourself; no manufacturer yet makes ice-cream this way.)

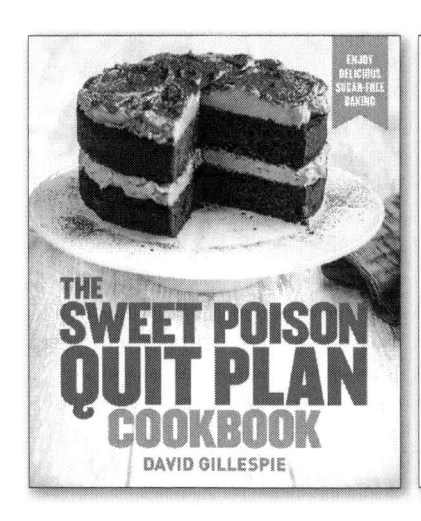

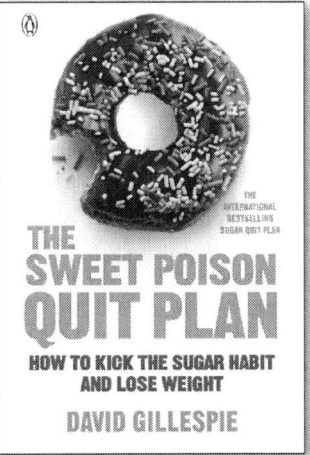

Yoghurts

I've presented this list in two formats so you can browse by sugar content or brand. You'll see that I've used a column called 'Adjusted Sugar'. This is a calculated amount based on removing the 4.7 grams of lactose that the typical yogurt contains. Lactose is a galactose molecule joined to a glucose molecule. The galactose molecule is metabolised to glucose by your liver and lactose is therefore essentially pure glucose and fructose free. Lactose does not count towards your 3g per 100g limit.

Yoghurts - by sugar content

Brand	Label	Adjusted % Sugar
Co Yo	Natural Coconut Milk Yogurt	0.0 %
Co Yo	Vanilla Coconut Milk Yogurt	0.0 %
Tesco	Free From Natural Soya Yogurt	0.0 %
Delamere Dairy	Plain Goats Yogurt	0.0 %
Alpro	Simply Plain Yogurt	0.0 %
Desi	Mild 'n' Tasty Yogurt	0.0 %
Benecol	Dairy Free Tropical Yogurt Drink	0.0 %
Liberté	Natural Greek Style Yogurt	0.0 %
St Helen's Farm	Fat Free Goats Milk Yogurt	0.0 %
St Helen's Farm	Natural Goats Milk Yogurt	0.0 %
Tesco	Cholesterol Reducing Blueberry Yogurt Drink	0.0 %
Danone	Actimel Fat Free Original Yogurt Drink	0.0 %
Morrisons	NuMe Fromage Frais	0.0 %
Tesco	Finest 0 % Fat Greek Yogurt	0.0 %
Tesco	Healthy Living 0 % Fat Fromage Frais Yogurt	0.0 %

Yoghurts – by sugar content (continued)

Brand	Label	Adjusted % Sugar
Danone	Actimel Fat Free Raspberry Yogurt Drink	0.0 %
Danone	Danio Natural Yogurt	0.0 %
Lancashire Farm	Live Whole Milk Natural Yogurt	0.0 %
Onken	Natural Set Low Fat Yoghurt	0.0 %
Tesco	Cholesterol Reducing Strawberry Yogurt Drink	0.0 %
Danone	Actimel Fat Free Strawberry Yogurt Drink	0.0 %
Onken	Natural Set Yoghurt	0.0 %
Irish Yogurts	Diet Indulgence Strawberry Cheesecake Fat Free Yogurt	0.0 %
Lancashire Farm	Natural Probiotic Yogurt	0.0 %
Tesco	Cholesterol Reducing Apricot & Peach Yogurt Drink	0.0 %
Fage	Total 2 % Greek Yoghurt	0.0 %
Fage	Total Classic Greek Yoghurt	0.0 %
Irish Yogurts	Diet Raspberry Fat Free Yogurt	0.0 %
Nomadic	Natural Ayran Yogurt Drink	0.0 %
Co Yo	Raw Chocolate Coconut Milk Yogurt	0.0 %
Henna	Natural Live Set Yogurt	0.0 %
Irish Yogurts	Diet Indulgence Tiramisu Fat Free Yogurt	0.0 %
Lancashire Farm	Low Fat Natural Probiotic Yogurt	0.0 %
ASDA	Extra Special Fat Free Greek Yogurt	0.0 %
ASDA	Extra Special Greek Yogurt	0.0 %
Fage	Total 0 % Greek Yoghurt	0.0 %
Irish Yogurts	Diet Passion Fruit Fat Free Yogurt	0.0 %
Onken	Natural Yoghurt	0.0 %

Yoghurts - by sugar content (continued)

Brand	Label	Adjusted % Sugar
Tesco	Finest Greek Yogurt	0.0 %
Irish Yogurts	Diet Indulgence Black Forrest Gateau Fat Free Yogurt	0.0 %
Sainsbury's	Normandy Natural Fat Free Fromage Frais	0.0 %
Irish Yogurts	Diet Blackcurrant Fat Free Yogurt	0.0 %
Irish Yogurts	Diet Blueberry Fat Free Yogurt	0.0 %
Irish Yogurts	Diet Indulgence Toffee Fat Free Yogurt	0.0 %
Irish Yogurts	Diet Mango & Lemon Fat Free Yogurt	0.0 %
Irish Yogurts	Low Fat Strawberry Greek Style Yogurt	0.0 %
Onken	Natural Fat Free Yoghurt	0.0 %
Irish Yogurts	Diet Peach Fat Free Yogurt	0.0 %
Co Yo	Pineapple Coconut Milk Yogurt	0.0 %
Flora	Pro.Active Original Yogurt Drink	0.0 %
Flora	Pro.Active Pomegranate & Raspberry Yogurt Drink	0.0 %
Flora	Pro.Active Strawberry Yogurt Drink	0.0 %
Glenisk	Organic Fat Free Natural Yogurt	0.0 %
Irish Yogurts	Diet Mandarin Fat Free Yogurt	0.0 %
Weight Watchers	Greek Style Natural Yogurt	0.0 %
Irish Yogurts	Diet Indulgence Apple & Cinnamon Fat Free Yogurt	0.0 %
Weight Watchers	Apricot & Nectarine Yogurt	0.0 %
Irish Yogurts	Diet Pineapple & Coconut Fat Free Yogurt	0.0 %
ASDA	Natural Set Yogurt	0.1 %
Irish Yogurts	Diet Indulgence Banoffee Fat Free Yogurt	0.1 %

Yoghurts – by sugar content (continued)

Brand	Label	Adjusted % Sugar
Woodlands Dairy	Natural Sheep Milk Yogurt	0.1 %
Woodlands Dairy	Organic Natural Sheep Milk Yogurt	0.1 %
ASDA	Fat Free Natural Fromage Frais	0.3 %
Flora	Pro.Active Mango & Cherry Yogurt Drink	0.3 %
Rachel's	Organic Natural Greek Style Yogurt	0.3 %
Irish Yogurts	Low Fat Pineapple & Coconut Greek Style Yogurt	0.4 %
Morrisons	Greek Style Yogurt	0.4 %
Sainsbury's	Greek Style Natural Yogurt	0.4 %
Tesco	Cholesterol Reducing Original Yogurt Drink	0.4 %
Weight Watchers	Layered Summer Fruit Fromage Frais	0.4 %
Co Yo	Mango Coconut Milk Yogurt	0.5 %
Co Yo	Mixed Berry Coconut Milk Yogurt	0.5 %
Sainsbury's	Fat Free Greek Style Natural Yogurt	0.5 %
Weight Watchers	Citrus Fruit Yogurt	0.5 %
Weight Watchers	Toffee & Vanilla Yogurt	0.5 %
ASDA	Greek Style Fat Free Yogurt	0.6 %
Glenisk	Organic Greek Style Natural Yogurt	0.6 %
Tesco	0 % Fat Greek Style Natural Yogurt	0.6 %
Weight Watchers	Greek Style Exotic Coconut Yogurt	0.6 %
Ella's Kitchen	Strawberry & Pear Yogurt	0.7 %
Tesco	Greek Style Natural Yogurt	0.7 %
Waitrose	Greek Style Natural Yogurt	0.7 %
Weight Watchers	Greek Style Honeyed Vanilla Yogurt	0.7 %
Weight Watchers	Layered Berry Fruit Fromage Frais	0.7 %

Yoghurts – by sugar content (continued)

Brand	Label	Adjusted % Sugar
Irish Yogurts	Diet Indulgence Rhubarb & Custard Fat Free Yogurt	0.8 %
Morrisons	Savers Low Fat Natural Yogurt	0.9 %
Yakult	Light Milk Drink	0.9 %
Benecol	Blueberry Yogurt Drink	1.0 %
Nomadic	Labneh Lebanese Style Yogurt	1.0 %
Benecol	Raspberry Yogurt Drink	1.1 %
Co Yo	Morello Cherry Coconut Milk Yogurt	1.2 %
Benecol	Plus Heart Vitamin B1 Yogurt Drink	1.3 %
Benecol	Strawberry Yogurt Drink	1.3 %
Glenisk	Natural Goats Milk Yogurt	1.3 %
Danone	Activia Natural Yogurt	1.4 %
Glenisk	Organic Whole Milk Natural Yogurt	1.4 %
Glenisk	Pure Original Blueberry Organic Yogurt	1.4 %
Glenisk	Pure Original Natural Organic Yogurt	1.4 %
Irish Yogurts	Creamier Champagne Rhubarb Live Yogurt	1.4 %
Irish Yogurts	Creamier Gooseberry Live Yogurt	1.4 %
Irish Yogurts	Creamier Pear & Plum Live Yogurt	1.4 %
Irish Yogurts	Creamier Strawberry & Vanilla Live Yogurt	1.4 %
Irish Yogurts	Diet Strawberry Fat Free Yogurt	1.4 %
Tesco	Healthy Living 0 % Fat Peach Yogurt	1.4 %
Benecol	Plus Bone Health Yogurt Drink	1.5 %
ASDA	Whole Milk Natural Yogurt	1.6 %
Danone	Shape 0 % Fat Rhubarb Crumble Yogurt	1.6 %
Danone	Shape 0 % Fat Strawberry Yogurt	1.6 %

Yoghurts - by sugar content (continued)

Brand	Label	Adjusted % Sugar
Glenisk	Pure Original Mango Organic Yogurt	1.6 %
Irish Yogurts	Diet Blackberry Fat Free Yogurt	1.6 %
Tesco	Healthy Living 0 % Fat Strawberry Yogurt	1.6 %
ASDA	Smart Price Low Fat Natural Yogurt	1.7 %
Muller	Light Cherry Yogurt	1.7 %
Sainsbury's	Fat Free Natural Yogurt	1.7 %
Waitrose	Fat Free Natural Yogurt	1.7 %
Woodlands Dairy	Natural Goats Milk Yogurt	1.7 %
Yeo Valley	Greek Style Natural Yogurt	1.7 %
Danone	Shape 0 % Fat Raspberry Yogurt	1.8 %
Morrisons	NuMe Fat Free Greek Style Yogurt	1.8 %
Sainsbury's	SO Organic Low Fat Natural Yogurt	1.8 %
Weight Watchers	Greek Style Luscious Lemon Yogurt	1.8 %
Yeo Valley	Natural Yogurt	1.8 %
ASDA	Greek Style Yogurt	1.9 %
Benecol	Peach & Apricot Yogurt Drink	1.9 %
Danone	Shape 0 % Fat Apple Crumble Yogurt	1.9 %
Irish Yogurts	Diet Pear & Mango Fat Free Yogurt	1.9 %
Sainsbury's	Natural Yogurt	1.9 %
Tesco	Whole Milk Natural Yogurt	1.9 %
Weight Watchers	Greek Style Sensational Strawberry Yogurt	1.9 %
Weight Watchers	Summer Fruit Yogurt	1.9 %
Danone	Shape 0 % Fat Peach & Passionfruit Yogurt	2.0 %
Glenisk	Organic Low Fat Natural Yogurt	2.1 %

Yoghurts - by sugar content (continued)

Brand	Label	Adjusted % Sugar
Irish Yogurts	Diet Natural Fat Free Yogurt	2.1 %
Tesco	Light Choices Natural Yogurt	2.1 %
Waitrose	Low Fat Natural Yogurt	2.1 %
Benecol	Light Yogurt Drink	2.2 %
Danone	Shape 0 % Fat Blackberry Yogurt	2.2 %
Danone	Shape 0 % Fat Cherry Yogurt	2.2 %
Irish Yogurts	Diet Apricot & Nectarine Fat Free Yogurt	2.2 %
Irish Yogurts	Diet Fruit of the Forest Fat Free Yogurt	2.2 %
Tesco	Low Fat Natural Yogurt	2.2 %
ASDA	Fat Free Rhubarb & Vanilla Yogurt	2.3 %
Danone	Shape 0 % Fat Apricot Yogurt	2.3 %
Danone	Shape 0 % Fat Pineapple & Coconut Yogurt	2.3 %
Muller	Light Coconut with a hint of Lime Yogurt	2.3 %
Muller	Light Organce & Dark Chocolate Yogurt	2.3 %
Muller	Light Vanilla Yogurt	2.3 %
Sainsbury's	Basics Low Fat Natural Yogurt	2.3 %
Tesco	Healthy Living 0 % Fat Vanilla Yogurt	2.3 %
Tesco	Low Fat Greek Style Natural Yogurt	2.3 %
Waitrose	Low Fat Greek Style Natural Yogurt	2.3 %
Yeo Valley	0 % Fat Greek Style Natural Yogurt	2.3 %
Longley Farm	Natural Yogurt	2.4 %
Muller	Light Peach & Pineapple Yogurt	2.4 %
Muller	Light Smooth Toffee Yogurt	2.4 %
Muller	Light Strawberry Yogurt	2.4 %

Yoghurts - by sugar content (continued)

Brand	Label	Adjusted % Sugar
Muller	Light Turkish Delight Yogurt	2.4 %
Muller	Light Vanilla & Dark Chocolate Yogurt	2.4 %
Sainsbury's	Low Fat Greek Style Natural Yogurt	2.4 %
Sainsbury's	Low Fat Natural Yogurt	2.4 %
Muller	Light Raspberry & Cranberry Yogurt	2.5 %
Tesco	Everyday Value Low Fat Natural Yogurt	2.5 %
ASDA	Fat Free Red Cherry Yogurt	2.6 %
ASDA	Greek Style Fat Free Peach Yogurt	2.6 %
Muller	Light Afterdinner Mint Yogurt	2.6 %
Muller	Light Rhubarb Yogurt	2.6 %
Glenisk	Organic 0 % Fat Yogurt with Granola	2.7 %
Longley Farm	BIO Natural Yogurt	2.7 %
Tesco	Healthy Living 0 % Fat Cherry Yogurt	2.7 %
ASDA	Fat Free Blueberry Yogurt	2.8 %
Morrisons	Low Fat Greek Style Yogurt	2.8 %
Danone	Activia Vanilla 0 % Fat Yogurt	2.9 %
Ella's Kitchen	Mango Fromage Frais	2.9 %
Muller	Light Mango & Passionfruit Yogurt	2.9 %
Tesco	Healthy Living 0 % Fat Toffee Yogurt	2.9 %
ASDA	Fat Free Natural Yogurt	3.0 %
ASDA	Greek Style Fat Free Vanilla Yogurt	3.0 %
Muller	Light Banana & Custard Yogurt	3.0 %
Muller	Light Mandarin Yogurt	3.0 %

Yoghurts - by brand

Brand	Label	Adjusted % Sugar
Alpro	Simply Plain Yogurt	0.0 %
ASDA	Extra Special Fat Free Greek Yogurt	0.0 %
	Extra Special Greek Yogurt	0.0 %
	Natural Set Yogurt	0.1 %
	Fat Free Natural Fromage Frais	0.3 %
	Greek Style Fat Free Yogurt	0.6 %
	Whole Milk Natural Yogurt	1.6 %
	Smart Price Low Fat Natural Yogurt	1.7 %
	Greek Style Yogurt	1.9 %
	Fat Free Rhubarb & Vanilla Yogurt	2.3 %
	Fat Free Red Cherry Yogurt	2.6 %
	Greek Style Fat Free Peach Yogurt	2.6 %
	Fat Free Blueberry Yogurt	2.8 %
	Fat Free Natural Yogurt	3.0 %
	Greek Style Fat Free Vanilla Yogurt	3.0 %
Benecol	Dairy Free Tropical Yogurt Drink	0.0 %
	Blueberry Yogurt Drink	1.0 %
	Raspberry Yogurt Drink	1.1 %
	Plus Heart Vitamin B1 Yogurt Drink	1.3 %
	Strawberry Yogurt Drink	1.3 %
	Plus Bone Health Yogurt Drink	1.5 %
	Peach & Apricot Yogurt Drink	1.9 %
	Light Yogurt Drink	2.2 %
Co Yo	Natural Coconut Milk Yogurt	0.0 %
	Vanilla Coconut Milk Yogurt	0.0 %
	Raw Chocolate Coconut Milk Yogurt	0.0 %

Yoghurts – by brand (continued)

Brand	Label	Adjusted % Sugar
Co Yo	Pineapple Coconut Milk Yogurt	0.0 %
	Mango Coconut Milk Yogurt	0.5 %
	Mixed Berry Coconut Milk Yogurt	0.5 %
	Morello Cherry Coconut Milk Yogurt	1.2 %
Danone	Actimel Fat Free Original Yogurt Drink	0.0 %
	Actimel Fat Free Raspberry Yogurt Drink	0.0 %
	Danio Natural Yogurt	0.0 %
	Actimel Fat Free Strawberry Yogurt Drink	0.0 %
	Activia Natural Yogurt	1.4 %
	Shape 0 % Fat Rhubarb Crumble Yogurt	1.6 %
	Shape 0 % Fat Strawberry Yogurt	1.6 %
	Shape 0 % Fat Raspberry Yogurt	1.8 %
	Shape 0 % Fat Apple Crumble Yogurt	1.9 %
	Shape 0 % Fat Peach & Passionfruit Yogurt	2.0 %
	Shape 0 % Fat Blackberry Yogurt	2.2 %
	Shape 0 % Fat Cherry Yogurt	2.2 %
	Shape 0 % Fat Apricot Yogurt	2.3 %
	Shape 0 % Fat Pineapple & Coconut Yogurt	2.3 %
	Activia Vanilla 0 % Fat Yogurt	2.9 %
Delamere Dairy	Plain Goats Yogurt	0.0 %
Desi	Mild 'n' Tasty Yogurt	0.0 %
Ella's Kitchen	Strawberry & Pear Yogurt	0.7 %
	Mango Fromage Frais	2.9 %
Fage	Total 2 % Greek Yoghurt	0.0 %

Yoghurts – by brand (continued)

Brand	Label	Adjusted % Sugar
Fage	Total Classic Greek Yoghurt	0.0 %
	Total 0 % Greek Yoghurt	0.0 %
Flora	Pro.Active Original Yogurt Drink	0.0 %
	Pro.Active Pomegranate & Raspberry Yogurt Drink	0.0 %
	Pro.Active Strawberry Yogurt Drink	0.0 %
	Pro.Active Mango & Cherry Yogurt Drink	0.3 %
Glenisk	Organic Fat Free Natural Yogurt	0.0 %
	Organic Greek Style Natural Yogurt	0.6 %
	Natural Goats Milk Yogurt	1.3 %
	Organic Whole Milk Natural Yogurt	1.4 %
	Pure Original Blueberry Organic Yogurt	1.4 %
	Pure Original Natural Organic Yogurt	1.4 %
	Pure Original Mango Organic Yogurt	1.6 %
	Organic Low Fat Natural Yogurt	2.1 %
	Organic 0 % Fat Yogurt with Granola	2.7 %
Henna	Natural Live Set Yogurt	0.0 %
Irish Yogurts	Diet Indulgence Strawberry Cheesecake Fat Free Yogurt	0.0 %
	Diet Raspberry Fat Free Yogurt	0.0 %
	Diet Indulgence Tiramisu Fat Free Yogurt	0.0 %
	Diet Passion Fruit Fat Free Yogurt	0.0 %
	Diet Indulgence Black Forrest Gateau Fat Free Yogurt	0.0 %
	Diet Blackcurrant Fat Free Yogurt	0.0 %
	Diet Blueberry Fat Free Yogurt	0.0 %
	Diet Indulgence Toffee Fat Free Yogurt	0.0 %

Yoghurts – by brand (continued)

Brand	Label	Adjusted % Sugar
Irish Yogurts	Diet Mango & Lemon Fat Free Yogurt	0.0 %
	Low Fat Strawberry Greek Style Yogurt	0.0 %
	Diet Peach Fat Free Yogurt	0.0 %
	Diet Mandarin Fat Free Yogurt	0.0 %
	Diet Indulgence Apple & Cinnamon Fat Free Yogurt	0.0 %
	Diet Pineapple & Coconut Fat Free Yogurt	0.0 %
	Diet Indulgence Banoffee Fat Free Yogurt	0.1 %
	Low Fat Pineapple & Coconut Greek Style Yogurt	0.4 %
	Diet Indulgence Rhubarb & Custard Fat Free Yogurt	0.8 %
	Creamier Champagne Rhubarb Live Yogurt	1.4 %
	Creamier Gooseberry Live Yogurt	1.4 %
	Creamier Pear & Plum Live Yogurt	1.4 %
	Creamier Strawberry & Vanilla Live Yogurt	1.4 %
	Diet Strawberry Fat Free Yogurt	1.4 %
	Diet Blackberry Fat Free Yogurt	1.6 %
	Diet Pear & Mango Fat Free Yogurt	1.9 %
	Diet Natural Fat Free Yogurt	2.1 %
	Diet Apricot & Nectarine Fat Free Yogurt	2.2 %
	Diet Fruit of the Forest Fat Free Yogurt	2.2 %
Lancashire Farm	Live Whole Milk Natural Yogurt	0.0 %
	Natural Probiotic Yogurt	0.0 %
	Low Fat Natural Probiotic Yogurt	0.0 %
Liberté	Natural Greek Style Yogurt	0.0 %

Yoghurts - by brand (continued)

Brand	Label	Adjusted % Sugar
Longley Farm	Natural Yogurt	2.4 %
	BIO Natural Yogurt	2.7 %
Morrisons	NuMe Fromage Frais	0.0 %
	Greek Style Yogurt	0.4 %
	Savers Low Fat Natural Yogurt	0.9 %
	NuMe Fat Free Greek Style Yogurt	1.8 %
	Low Fat Greek Style Yogurt	2.8 %
Muller	Light Cherry Yogurt	1.7 %
	Light Coconut with a hint of Lime Yogurt	2.3 %
	Light Organce & Dark Chocolate Yogurt	2.3 %
	Light Vanilla Yogurt	2.3 %
	Light Peach & Pineapple Yogurt	2.4 %
	Light Smooth Toffee Yogurt	2.4 %
	Light Strawberry Yogurt	2.4 %
	Light Turkish Delight Yogurt	2.4 %
	Light Vanilla & Dark Chocolate Yogurt	2.4 %
	Light Raspberry & Cranberry Yogurt	2.5 %
	Light Afterdinner Mint Yogurt	2.6 %
	Light Rhubarb Yogurt	2.6 %
	Light Mango & Passionfruit Yogurt	2.9 %
	Light Banana & Custard Yogurt	3.0 %
	Light Mandarin Yogurt	3.0 %
Nomadic	Natural Ayran Yogurt Drink	0.0 %
	Labneh Lebanese Style Yogurt	1.0 %
Onken	Natural Set Low Fat Yoghurt	0.0 %

Yoghurts – by brand (continued)

Brand	Label	Adjusted % Sugar
Onken	Natural Set Yoghurt	0.0 %
	Natural Yoghurt	0.0 %
	Natural Fat Free Yoghurt	0.0 %
Rachel's	Organic Natural Greek Style Yogurt	0.3 %
Sainsbury's	Normandy Natural Fat Free Fromage Frais	0.0 %
	Greek Style Natural Yogurt	0.4 %
	Fat Free Greek Style Natural Yogurt	0.5 %
	Fat Free Natural Yogurt	1.7 %
	SO Organic Low Fat Natural Yogurt	1.8 %
	Natural Yogurt	1.9 %
	Basics Low Fat Natural Yogurt	2.3 %
	Low Fat Greek Style Natural Yogurt	2.4 %
	Low Fat Natural Yogurt	2.4 %
St Helen's Farm	Fat Free Goats Milk Yogurt	0.0 %
	Natural Goats Milk Yogurt	0.0 %
Tesco	Free From Natural Soya Yogurt	0.0 %
	Cholesterol Reducing Blueberry Yogurt Drink	0.0 %
	Finest 0 % Fat Greek Yogurt	0.0 %
	Healthy Living 0 % Fat Fromage Frais Yogurt	0.0 %
	Cholesterol Reducing Strawberry Yogurt Drink	0.0 %
	Cholesterol Reducing Apricot & Peach Yogurt Drink	0.0 %
	Finest Greek Yogurt	0.0 %
	Cholesterol Reducing Original Yogurt Drink	0.4 %
	0 % Fat Greek Style Natural Yogurt	0.6 %

Yoghurts – by brand (continued)

Brand	Label	Adjusted % Sugar
Tesco	Greek Style Natural Yogurt	0.7 %
	Healthy Living 0 % Fat Peach Yogurt	1.4 %
	Healthy Living 0 % Fat Strawberry Yogurt	1.6 %
	Whole Milk Natural Yogurt	1.9 %
	Light Choices Natural Yogurt	2.1 %
	Low Fat Natural Yogurt	2.2 %
	Healthy Living 0 % Fat Vanilla Yogurt	2.3 %
	Low Fat Greek Style Natural Yogurt	2.3 %
	Everyday Value Low Fat Natural Yogurt	2.5 %
	Healthy Living 0 % Fat Cherry Yogurt	2.7 %
	Healthy Living 0 % Fat Toffee Yogurt	2.9 %
Waitrose	Greek Style Natural Yogurt	0.7 %
	Fat Free Natural Yogurt	1.7 %
	Low Fat Natural Yogurt	2.1 %
	Low Fat Greek Style Natural Yogurt	2.3 %
Weight Watchers	Greek Style Natural Yogurt	0.0 %
	Apricot & Nectarine Yogurt	0.0 %
	Layered Summer Fruit Fromage Frais	0.4 %
	Citrus Fruit Yogurt	0.5 %
	Toffee & Vanilla Yogurt	0.5 %
	Greek Style Exotic Coconut Yogurt	0.6 %
	Greek Style Honeyed Vanilla Yogurt	0.7 %
	Layered Berry Fruit Fromage Frais	0.7 %
	Greek Style Luscious Lemon Yogurt	1.8 %
	Greek Style Sensational Strawberry Yogurt	1.9 %

Yoghurts - by brand (continued)

Brand	Label	Adjusted % Sugar
Weight Watchers	Summer Fruit Yogurt	1.9 %
Woodlands Dairy	Natural Sheep Milk Yogurt	0.1 %
	Organic Natural Sheep Milk Yogurt	0.1 %
	Natural Goats Milk Yogurt	1.7 %
Yakult	Light Milk Drink	0.9 %
Yeo Valley	Greek Style Natural Yogurt	1.7 %
	Natural Yogurt	1.8 %
	0 % Fat Greek Style Natural Yogurt	2.3 %

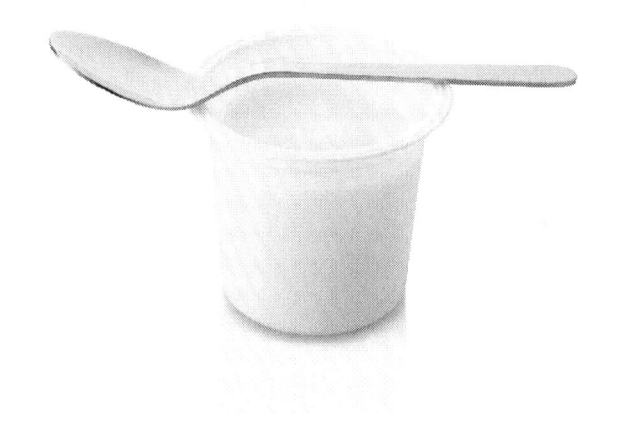

Breads

I've presented this list in two formats so you can browse by sugar content or brand. Almost all of the supermarket brands of bread contain rapeseed oil or another seed oil. If you are concerned about seed oil content then you will need to read the labels carefully. *Avoid any that say they contain 'Vegetable Oil'*

Breads - by sugar content

Brand	Label	% Sugar
Amisa Organic	Gluten Free Focaccia Rolls	0.0 %
Dawn Bread	Plain Paratha	0.0 %
The Polish Bakery	Rye 100 %	0.0 %
Tesco	Traditional Spanish Tortilla	0.5 %
Waitrose	Stonebaked Ficelle Bread	0.5 %
Bfree	Soft White Loaf	0.6 %
Bfree	Plain Bagel	0.7 %
ASDA	Free From White Sliced Loaf	0.8 %
Pacificio Italiano	Olive Ciabatta	0.8 %
Tesco	Six Grain Loaf	0.8 %
Kelderman	German Style Rye Bread	0.9 %
Biona Organic	Rice Wholegrain Gluten Free Bread	1.0 %
Cranks	Whole Lotta Loaf Bread	1.0 %
Irwin's	Irish Soda Bread Minis	1.0 %
Irwin's	Soda Farls	1.0 %
Newburn Bakehouse	White Farmhouse Loaf	1.0 %
The Polish Bakery	Dark Rye Bread with Inulin	1.0 %
Waitrose	Essential Cheese & Garlic Tear & Share Bread	1.0 %

Breads - by sugar content (continued)

Brand	Label	% Sugar
Waitrose	Stonebaked Spelt Bread	1.0 %
Waitrose	White Baguette	1.0 %
ASDA	Chosen by Kids Crumpets	1.1 %
ASDA	Large White Pittas	1.1 %
ASDA	White Pittas	1.1 %
Lakeland Bake	Squmpets	1.1 %
Lakeland Bake	Teddy Bear Crumpets	1.1 %
Newburn Bakehouse	Brown Farmhouse Loaf	1.1 %
Pacificio Italiano	Half Ciabatta	1.1 %
Pacificio Italiano	Plain Ciabatta	1.1 %
Udi's	White Sandwich Bread	1.1 %
Waitrose	Petit Pain	1.1 %
ASDA	Crumpet Squares	1.2 %
Lakeland Bake	Traditional Crumpets	1.2 %
Newburn Bakehouse	Soft Seeded Rolls	1.2 %
Tesco	Bakery Seeded Panini	1.2 %
Tesco	Bakery Three Cheese Bread	1.2 %
The Polish Bakery	Half Rye Half Wheat Bread	1.2 %
The Polish Bakery	Polish Style Caraway Seed Bread	1.2 %
The Polish Bakery	Poppy Seed Bread	1.2 %
Waitrose	Grand Rustic Bread	1.2 %
Waitrose	Pain Rustica Bread	1.2 %
ASDA	Seed & Oatmeal Pittas	1.3 %
Genius	Brown Rolls	1.3 %

Breads - by sugar content (continued)

Brand	Label	% Sugar
Kingsmill	50/50 Pockets	1.3 %
Newburn Bakehouse	Soft White Rolls	1.3 %
Old El Paso	Wholewheat Tortillas	1.3 %
Tesco	Bakery Cheese Topped Sub	1.3 %
Tesco	Kalamata Olive Bloomer	1.3 %
Dina	White Pitta Bread	1.4 %
DS Gluten Free	White Rolls	1.4 %
Newburn Bakehouse	Seeded Farmhouse Loaf	1.4 %
Ocado	Seeded Wraps	1.4 %
Sainsbury's	Be Good Plain Mini Naan	1.4 %
Waitrose	Love Life Stoneground Wholemeal Loaf	1.4 %
Weight Watchers	Love Fibre Wraps	1.4 %
Irwin's	Softee White Rolls	1.5 %
Morrisons	Signature White Farmhouse Loaf	1.5 %
Sainsbury's	Taste the Difference Garlic & Coriander Naan Bread	1.5 %
Tesco	Bakery Chunky Cheese Roll	1.5 %
Tesco	Bakery Tiger Roll	1.5 %
Tesco	Mediterranean Herb Pitta Squares	1.5 %
Tesco	White Pitta	1.5 %
The Polish Bakery	Brown Bread	1.5 %
The Polish Bakery	Sunflower Seed Bread	1.5 %
Weight Watchers	Petit Pains	1.5 %
Amisa Organic	Gluten Free Vitality Breakfast Rolls	1.6 %
Lakeland Bake	Just made for you Toaster Crumpets	1.6 %

Breads - by sugar content (continued)

Brand	Label	% Sugar
Sainsbury's	Flamebaked Chapatti	1.6 %
Sainsbury's	Flamebaked Garlic & Coriander Naan	1.6 %
Tesco	Bakery Sour Dough Bloomer	1.6 %
Tesco	Finest Garlic & Coriander Naan Bread	1.6 %
The Polish Bakery	Granny's Sesame Seed Bread	1.6 %
Waitrose	Roasted Garlic Ciabatta	1.6 %
ASDA	Finger Crumpets	1.7 %
ASDA	Garlic & Coriander Pittas	1.7 %
Bfree	Soft White Rolls	1.7 %
Dina	Golden Naan	1.7 %
Dina	Wholemeal Pitta Bread	1.7 %
Kingsmill	White Pockets	1.7 %
Waitrose	Farmhouse Wholemeal Loaf	1.7 %
Waitrose	Love Life Gluten Free Seeded Loaf	1.7 %
Waitrose	Wholemeal Long Tin Loaf	1.7 %
Warburtons	Soft House Farmhouse	1.7 %
ASDA	Large Wholemeal Pittas	1.8 %
ASDA	White Tortillas	1.8 %
ASDA	Wholemeal Pittas	1.8 %
Irwin's	Brown Rolls	1.8 %
Irwin's	Softee Loaf	1.8 %
Lakeland Bake	Wholemeal Crumpets	1.8 %
Morrisons	M Kitchen Indian Takeaway Chapatti	1.8 %
Sainsbury's	Flamebaked Plain Naan	1.8 %
Sainsbury's	Taste the Difference Crumpets	1.8 %
Tesco	Bakery Ploughmans Cob	1.8 %

Breads - by sugar content (continued)

Brand	Label	% Sugar
Tesco	Finest Plain Naan Bread	1.8 %
Tesco	Reduced Fat Plain Naan	1.8 %
Tesco	Wholemeal Pitta Squares	1.8 %
Waitrose	Organic Brown Loaf	1.8 %
Biona Organic	Buckwheat Rice Wholegrain Gluten Free Bread	1.9 %
Biona Organic	Golden Linseed Omega 3 Rye Bread	1.9 %
Lakeland Bake	Mature Cheddar Cheese Crumpets	1.9 %
Morrisons	M Kitchen Indian Takeaway Plain Naan	1.9 %
Old El Paso	Stand 'n' Stuff Soft Flour Tortillas	1.9 %
Tesco	Stay Fresh White Bread	1.9 %
Waitrose	Love Life Wholemeal & Seeds Bread	1.9 %
Waitrose	Mixed Seeds Baguette	1.9 %
Biona Organic	Millet Wholegrain Gluten Free Bread	2.0 %
Biona Organic	Rice & Sunflower Wholegrain Gluten Free Bread	2.0 %
Genius	Soft Brown Sandwich Bread	2.0 %
Lakeland Bake	Buttermilk Crumpets	2.0 %
Morrisons	M Kitchen Indian Takeaway Garlic & Coriander Naan	2.0 %
Old El Paso	Large Flour Tortillas	2.0 %
Robert's Bakery	White Rolls	2.0 %
Sainsbury's	Chapattis	2.0 %
Santa Maria	Corn & Wheat Soft Tortillas	2.0 %
Tesco	Bakery Panini	2.0 %
Tesco	Everyday Value Plain Naan Breads	2.0 %
Tesco	White Pitta Squares	2.0 %

Breads - by sugar content (continued)

Brand	Label	% Sugar
The Food Doctor	Multi Seed & Cereal Pittas	2.0 %
Waitrose	Six Seeded Brown Batch Bread	2.0 %
Warburtons	Thick & Fluffy Crumpets	2.0 %
ASDA	2 Plain Naans	2.1 %
Irwin's	High Fibre Loaf	2.1 %
Kingsmill	Soft White Rolls	2.1 %
Morrisons	Just For Kids Wheat & White Wraps	2.1 %
Sainsbury's	Soft Flour Tortillas	2.1 %
Waitrose	Heyford Wholemeal Bread	2.1 %
Waitrose	Love Life Gluten Free White Pitta	2.1 %
Waitrose	Stonebaked Boule	2.1 %
Biona Organic	Pumpkin Seed Rye Bread	2.2 %
Genius	Original White Bread	2.2 %
Genius	Soft Rolls	2.2 %
Hovis	Nimble Wholemeal	2.2 %
Irwin's	High Fibre Irish Batch Loaf	2.2 %
Kingsmill	50/50 Muffins	2.2 %
Kingsmill	Square Crumpets	2.2 %
Robert's Bakery	White Danish Loaf	2.2 %
Robert's Bakery	White Farmhouse Loaf	2.2 %
Sainsbury's	Be Good Plain Wraps	2.2 %
Sainsbury's	Chilli & Garlic Naan	2.2 %
Sharwood's	Garlic & Coriander Mini Naans	2.2 %
Tesco	Finest Ciabatta	2.2 %
Tesco	Panini Rolls	2.2 %
Tesco	Plain Tortilla Wraps	2.2 %

Breads - by sugar content (continued)

Brand	Label	% Sugar
Tesco	Stay Fresh Wholemeal Bread	2.2 %
Waitrose	Stonebaked Baguette	2.2 %
Warburtons	White Loaf	2.2 %
Weight Watchers	Soft Brown Danish	2.2 %
Bfree	Brown Seeded Rolls	2.3 %
Cranks	Breaditerranean Bread	2.3 %
Cranks	Hippity Homity Bread	2.3 %
Dina	White Bread Wraps	2.3 %
Hollyland Bakery	Wholemeal Pitta	2.3 %
Irwin's	7 Seeded Wholemeal Loaf	2.3 %
Morrisons	Baked by us Cheddar Cheese Muffin	2.3 %
Robert's Bakery	Thick White Loaf	2.3 %
Robert's Bakery	White Sourdough	2.3 %
Robert's Bakery	Wholemeal Loaf	2.3 %
Sainsbury's	Garlic & Coriander Naans	2.3 %
Sainsbury's	SO Organic Sunflower & Pumpkin Seed Bread	2.3 %
Tesco	Stonebaked Ciabatta	2.3 %
The Food Doctor	Multi Seed & Cereal Loaf	2.3 %
Waitrose	Essential Plain Tortilla Wraps	2.3 %
Waitrose	Essential Wholemeal Tortillas Wraps	2.3 %
Waitrose	Paysan Rustica Bread	2.3 %
Waitrose	Roasted Garlic Flatbread	2.3 %
Warburtons	Crusty White Loaf	2.3 %
Warburtons	Danish White Loaf	2.3 %
Warburtons	Sliced White Rolls	2.3 %

Breads - by sugar content (continued)

Brand	Label	% Sugar
Weight Watchers	Garlic & Coriander Mini Naans	2.3 %
ASDA	Seeded Tortillas	2.4 %
ASDA	White & Wheat Tortillas	2.4 %
Biona Organic	Vitality Sprouted Seeds Rye Bread	2.4 %
Cranks	Carry on Carrot Bread	2.4 %
Hollyland Bakery	White Pitta	2.4 %
Hovis	Granary Wholemeal	2.4 %
Morrisons	Baked by Us Mini Garlic & Coriander Naan Bread	2.4 %
Morrisons	White Pitta	2.4 %
Morrisons	White Pitta Dippers	2.4 %
Robert's Bakery	Floury Rolls	2.4 %
Tesco	70 Calorie Wholemeal Bread	2.4 %
Tesco	Bakery Ciabatta Roll	2.4 %
Udi's	Brown Sandwich Bread	2.4 %
Waitrose	Essential Garlic Baguette	2.4 %
Waitrose	White Flute Bread	2.4 %
Warburtons	Half & Half Loaf	2.4 %
Warburtons	Wholemeal Loaf	2.4 %
Weight Watchers	Plain Mini Naans	2.4 %
ASDA	Free From Garlic & Coriander Naan Breads	2.5 %
Bfree	Brown Seeded Loaf	2.5 %
Bfree	Multiseed Bagel	2.5 %
Genius	Triple Seeded Sandwich Bread	2.5 %
Hovis	Best of Both Rolls	2.5 %

Breads - by sugar content (continued)

Brand	Label	% Sugar
Hovis	Granary Original Rolls	2.5 %
Kingsmill	50/50 Rolls	2.5 %
Morrisons	Baked by us All Butter Muffin	2.5 %
Ocado	White Pitta	2.5 %
Old El Paso	Regular Flour Tortillas	2.5 %
Patak's	Plain Chapattis	2.5 %
Robert's Bakery	50 % White 50 % Wholemeal Loaf	2.5 %
Sainsbury's	Plain Tortilla Wraps	2.5 %
Sainsbury's	Wholemeal Tortillas Wraps	2.5 %
Sharwood's	Plain Chapattis	2.5 %
Tesco	Bakery Organic White Bloomer	2.5 %
Tesco	Takeaway Plain Mega Naan	2.5 %
Tesco	Wholemeal Pitta	2.5 %
Waitrose	Essential Picnic White Pitta	2.5 %
Waitrose	Grand Mange Paysan	2.5 %
Waitrose	Mixed Olive Ficelle Bread	2.5 %
Waitrose	Sourdough with Seeds Baguette	2.5 %
ASDA	White Mini Wraps	2.6 %
Dina	Tannour Thin Wraps	2.6 %
Genius	Crumpets	2.6 %
Irwin's	Multigrain Brown Pan Loaf	2.6 %
Morrisons	White Tortilla Wraps	2.6 %
Robert's Bakery	Tiger Bloomer	2.6 %
Robert's Bakery	White Finger Rolls	2.6 %
Sainsbury's	Panini Rolls	2.6 %
Sainsbury's	Plain Naans	2.6 %

Breads – by sugar content (continued)

Brand	Label	% Sugar
Tesco	Bakery Crusty White Roll	2.6 %
Tesco	Bakery Organic Brown Bloomer	2.6 %
Tesco	Cheese & Garlic Flatbread	2.6 %
Tesco	Light Choices Mini Naan Bread	2.6 %
Tesco	Mediterranean Herb Tortilla Wraps	2.6 %
Tesco	Toastie White Bread	2.6 %
Udi's	Tiger Bloomer	2.6 %
Waitrose	Grand Mange Blanc	2.6 %
Waitrose	Poppy Seed Roll	2.6 %
Warburtons	Old English White	2.6 %
Warburtons	Seeded Batch Loaf	2.6 %
Weight Watchers	Soft Malted Danish	2.6 %
Weight Watchers	Thick Sliced Wholemeal	2.6 %
ASDA	Bakers Gold Wholemeal	2.7 %
ASDA	Garlic & Coriander Naans	2.7 %
ASDA	Garlic Tortilla Wraps	2.7 %
ASDA	Garlic Tortilla Wraps	2.7 %
ASDA	Plain Chapattis	2.7 %
Dietary Specials	White Ciabatta Rolls	2.7 %
DS Gluten Free	White Ciabatta Rolls	2.7 %
Genius	Triple Seeded Rolls	2.7 %
Hovis	Hearty Oats	2.7 %
Hovis	Nimble Malted Wholegrain	2.7 %
Irwin's	Irish Batch Loaf	2.7 %
Irwin's	Nutty Crust Loaf	2.7 %
Irwin's	White Rolls	2.7 %

Breads – by sugar content (continued)

Brand	Label	% Sugar
Morrisons	Garlic & Coriander Naan Bread	2.7 %
Ocado	Bake at Home White Baguettes	2.7 %
Ocado	Bake at Home White Petit Pains	2.7 %
Ocado	Chilli Wraps	2.7 %
Ocado	Plain Wraps	2.7 %
Robert's Bakery	Seeded Farmhouse	2.7 %
Sainsbury's	SO Organic Seeded Wholemeal Rolls	2.7 %
Santa Maria	Wholemeal Soft Tortillas	2.7 %
Shana	Original Paratha	2.7 %
Tesco	Bakery Cheese Topped Roll	2.7 %
Tesco	Finest Stone Ground Wholemeal Farmhouse Bread	2.7 %
Udi's	Classic Finger Rolls	2.7 %
Waitrose	Organic Farmhouse Wholegrain Loaf	2.7 %
Weight Watchers	Garlic & Herb Ciabatta	2.7 %
Weight Watchers	Garlic & Herb Petit Pains	2.7 %
Weight Watchers	Soft White Danish	2.7 %
ASDA	Wholemeal Finger Rolls	2.8 %
ASDA	Wholemeal Tortillas	2.8 %
Dina	Chapattis	2.8 %
DS Gluten Free	Wholesome Seeded Sliced Loaf	2.8 %
Hollyland Bakery	White Khobez	2.8 %
Loyd Grossman	Garlic & Coriander Naan Breads	2.8 %
Loyd Grossman	Plain Naan Breads	2.8 %
Morrisons	Bake at Home Ciabatta Rolls	2.8 %
Morrisons	White Loaf	2.8 %

Breads - by sugar content (continued)

Brand	Label	% Sugar
Morrisons	Wholemeal Loaf	2.8 %
Newburn Bakehouse	White Baguettes	2.8 %
Old El Paso	Mini Flour Tortillas	2.8 %
Robert's Bakery	Soft White Deli Rolls	2.8 %
Sainsbury's	Basics White Pitta	2.8 %
Sainsbury's	Taste the Difference Wholemeal Bloomers	2.8 %
Tesco	Bakery Sesame Roll	2.8 %
Tesco	Bakery Soft Sub	2.8 %
Tesco	Everyday Value White Pitta Bread	2.8 %
Tesco	Finest Cornish All Butter Toasting Muffins	2.8 %
Tesco	Seeded Burger Buns	2.8 %
Tesco	Seeded Tortilla Wraps	2.8 %
Waitrose	Indian Plain Parathas	2.8 %
Waitrose	Love Life Farmhouse Batch Wholemeal Loaf	2.8 %
Waitrose	Pain au Levain	2.8 %
Waitrose	White with Wholemeal Loaf	2.8 %
Warburtons	Wholemeal Rolls	2.8 %
Allinson	Wholemeal Sliced Loaf	2.9 %
Biona Organic	Chia & Flax Seed Rye Bread	2.9 %
Biona Organic	Sunflower Seed Rye Bread	2.9 %
Country Miller	Wholemeal Seeded Bloomer	2.9 %
Dina	Garlic & Coriander Naan	2.9 %
Irwin's	High Fibre Nutty Crust Loaf	2.9 %
Kingsmill	Crusts Away 50/50 Bread	2.9 %

Breads - by sugar content (continued)

Brand	Label	% Sugar
Loyd Grossman	Chapattis	2.9 %
Morrisons	Wholemeal Pitta	2.9 %
Patak's	Plain Naans	2.9 %
Robert's Bakery	Soft Brown Loaf	2.9 %
Sainsbury's	Flamebaked Garlic & Parsley Flatbread	2.9 %
Tesco	Bakery Salt & Pepper Bloomer	2.9 %
Tesco	Bakery Tiger Cheese Bloomer	2.9 %
Tesco	Plain Naan	2.9 %
Vogels	Sunflower & Barley	2.9 %
Waitrose	Essential Mini White Pitta	2.9 %
Warburtons	Large White Rolls	2.9 %
Warburtons	Tear & Toast Muffins	2.9 %
Warburtons	White Sub Rolls	2.9 %
Allinson	Sunflower & Pumpkin Sliced Loaf	3.0 %
Amisa Organic	Gluten Free Flax Seed Rice Bread	3.0 %
ASDA	Buckwheat & Poppy Seed	3.0 %
Baltona	Artisan Brown Bread	3.0 %
Hovis	Wholemeal Rolls	3.0 %
Kingsmill	Crumpets	3.0 %
Kingsmill	Great White Bread	3.0 %
Morrisons	Bake at Home Bread	3.0 %
Morrisons	Plain Naans	3.0 %
Morrisons	Savers Part Baked White Baguettes	3.0 %
Ocado	Large Wholemeal Tin Loaf	3.0 %
Patak's	Garlic & Coriander Naans	3.0 %
Sainsbury's	Oat Topped Wholemeal Deli Rolls	3.0 %

Breads - by sugar content (continued)

Brand	Label	% Sugar
Sainsbury's	SO Organic Multiseeded Wholemeal Bread	3.0 %
Shana	Garlic Paratha	3.0 %
Tesco	Bakery Cheese Topped Baton	3.0 %
Tesco	Bakery Corn Bread	3.0 %
Tesco	Bakery Poppy Seed Bloomer	3.0 %
Tesco	Bakery Rye Bread	3.0 %
Tesco	Everyday Value Crumpets	3.0 %
Tesco	Wholemeal Farmhouse Bread	3.0 %
Waitrose	Love Life Farmhouse Wholemeal & Pumpkin Loaf	3.0 %
Waitrose	Love Life Wholemeal, Rye & Toasted Rye Grain Loaf	3.0 %
Warburtons	Soft White Pitta Halves	3.0 %

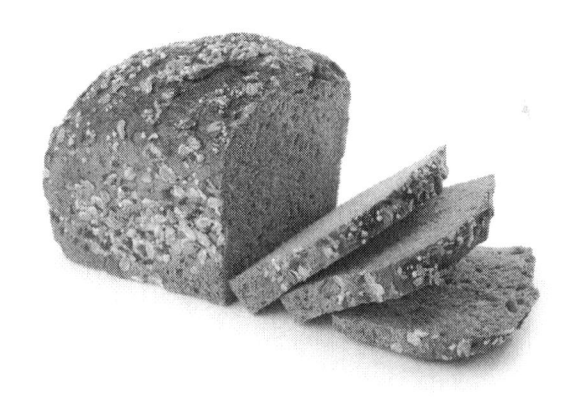

Breads - by brand

Brand	Label	% Sugar
Allinson	Wholemeal Sliced Loaf	2.9 %
	Sunflower & Pumpkin Sliced Loaf	3.0 %
Amisa Organic	Gluten Free Focaccia Rolls	0.0 %
	Gluten Free Vitality Breakfast Rolls	1.6 %
	Gluten Free Flax Seed Rice Bread	3.0 %
ASDA	Free From White Sliced Loaf	0.8 %
	Chosen by Kids Crumpets	1.1 %
	Large White Pittas	1.1 %
	White Pittas	1.1 %
	Crumpet Squares	1.2 %
	Seed & Oatmeal Pittas	1.3 %
	Finger Crumpets	1.7 %
	Garlic & Coriander Pittas	1.7 %
	Large Wholemeal Pittas	1.8 %
	White Tortillas	1.8 %
	Wholemeal Pittas	1.8 %
	2 Plain Naans	2.1 %
	Seeded Tortillas	2.4 %
	White & Wheat Tortillas	2.4 %
	Free From Garlic & Coriander Naan Breads	2.5 %
	White Mini Wraps	2.6 %
	Bakers Gold Wholemeal	2.7 %
	Garlic & Coriander Naans	2.7 %
	Garlic Tortilla Wraps	2.7 %
	Garlic Tortilla Wraps	2.7 %

Breads - by brand (continued)

Brand	Label	% Sugar
ASDA	Plain Chapattis	2.7 %
	Wholemeal Finger Rolls	2.8 %
	Wholemeal Tortillas	2.8 %
	Buckwheat & Poppy Seed	3.0 %
Baltona	Artisan Brown Bread	3.0 %
Bfree	Soft White Loaf	0.6 %
	Plain Bagel	0.7 %
	Soft White Rolls	1.7 %
	Brown Seeded Rolls	2.3 %
	Brown Seeded Loaf	2.5 %
	Multiseed Bagel	2.5 %
Biona Organic	Rice Wholegrain Gluten Free Bread	1.0 %
	Buckwheat Rice Wholegrain Gluten Free Bread	1.9 %
	Golden Linseed Omega 3 Rye Bread	1.9 %
	Millet Wholegrain Gluten Free Bread	2.0 %
	Rice & Sunflower Wholegrain Gluten Free Bread	2.0 %
	Pumpkin Seed Rye Bread	2.2 %
	Vitality Sprouted Seeds Rye Bread	2.4 %
	Chia & Flax Seed Rye Bread	2.9 %
	Sunflower Seed Rye Bread	2.9 %
Country Miller	Wholemeal Seeded Bloomer	2.9 %
Cranks	Whole Lotta Loaf Bread	1.0 %
	Breaditerranean Bread	2.3 %
	Hippity Homity Bread	2.3 %

Breads - by brand (continued)

Brand	Label	% Sugar
Cranks	Carry on Carrot Bread	2.4 %
Dawn Bread	Plain Paratha	0.0 %
Dietary Specials	White Ciabatta Rolls	2.7 %
Dina	White Pitta Bread	1.4 %
	Golden Naan	1.7 %
	Wholemeal Pitta Bread	1.7 %
	White Bread Wraps	2.3 %
	Tannour Thin Wraps	2.6 %
	Chapattis	2.8 %
	Garlic & Coriander Naan	2.9 %
DS Gluten Free	White Rolls	1.4 %
	White Ciabatta Rolls	2.7 %
	Wholesome Seeded Sliced Loaf	2.8 %
Genius	Brown Rolls	1.3 %
	Soft Brown Sandwich Bread	2.0 %
	Original White Bread	2.2 %
	Soft Rolls	2.2 %
	Triple Seeded Sandwich Bread	2.5 %
	Crumpets	2.6 %
	Triple Seeded Rolls	2.7 %
Hollyland Bakery	Wholemeal Pitta	2.3 %
	White Pitta	2.4 %
	White Khobez	2.8 %
Hovis	Nimble Wholemeal	2.2 %
	Granary Wholemeal	2.4 %
	Best of Both Rolls	2.5 %

Breads - by brand (continued)

Brand	Label	% Sugar
Hovis	Granary Original Rolls	2.5 %
	Hearty Oats	2.7 %
	Nimble Malted Wholegrain	2.7 %
	Wholemeal Rolls	3.0 %
Irwin's	Irish Soda Bread Minis	1.0 %
	Soda Farls	1.0 %
	Softee White Rolls	1.5 %
	Brown Rolls	1.8 %
	Softee Loaf	1.8 %
	High Fibre Loaf	2.1 %
	High Fibre Irish Batch Loaf	2.2 %
	7 Seeded Wholemeal Loaf	2.3 %
	Multigrain Brown Pan Loaf	2.6 %
	Irish Batch Loaf	2.7 %
	Nutty Crust Loaf	2.7 %
	White Rolls	2.7 %
	High Fibre Nutty Crust Loaf	2.9 %
Kelderman	German Style Rye Bread	0.9 %
Kingsmill	50/50 Pockets	1.3 %
	White Pockets	1.7 %
	Soft White Rolls	2.1 %
	50/50 Muffins	2.2 %
	Square Crumpets	2.2 %
	50/50 Rolls	2.5 %
	Crusts Away 50/50 Bread	2.9 %
	Crumpets	3.0 %

Breads - by brand (continued)

Brand	Label	% Sugar
Kingsmill	Great White Bread	3.0 %
Lakeland Bake	Squmpets	1.1 %
	Teddy Bear Crumpets	1.1 %
	Traditional Crumpets	1.2 %
	Just made for you Toaster Crumpets	1.6 %
	Wholemeal Crumpets	1.8 %
	Mature Cheddar Cheese Crumpets	1.9 %
	Buttermilk Crumpets	2.0 %
Loyd Grossman	Garlic & Coriander Naan Breads	2.8 %
	Plain Naan Breads	2.8 %
	Chapattis	2.9 %
Morrisons	Signature White Farmhouse Loaf	1.5 %
	M Kitchen Indian Takeaway Chapatti	1.8 %
	M Kitchen Indian Takeaway Plain Naan	1.9 %
	M Kitchen Indian Takeaway Garlic & Coriander Naan	2.0 %
	Just For Kids Wheat & White Wraps	2.1 %
	Baked by us Cheddar Cheese Muffin	2.3 %
	Baked by Us Mini Garlic & Coriander Naan Bread	2.4 %
	White Pitta	2.4 %
	White Pitta Dippers	2.4 %
	Baked by us All Butter Muffin	2.5 %
	White Tortilla Wraps	2.6 %
	Garlic & Coriander Naan Bread	2.7 %
	Bake at Home Ciabatta Rolls	2.8 %

Breads – by brand (continued)

Brand	Label	% Sugar
Morrisons	White Loaf	2.8 %
	Wholemeal Loaf	2.8 %
	Wholemeal Pitta	2.9 %
	Bake at Home Bread	3.0 %
	Plain Naans	3.0 %
	Savers Part Baked White Baguettes	3.0 %
Newburn Bakehouse	White Farmhouse Loaf	1.0 %
	Brown Farmhouse Loaf	1.1 %
	Soft Seeded Rolls	1.2 %
	Soft White Rolls	1.3 %
	Seeded Farmhouse Loaf	1.4 %
	White Baguettes	2.8 %
Ocado	Seeded Wraps	1.4 %
	White Pitta	2.5 %
	Bake at Home White Baguettes	2.7 %
	Bake at Home White Petit Pains	2.7 %
	Chilli Wraps	2.7 %
	Plain Wraps	2.7 %
	Large Wholemeal Tin Loaf	3.0 %
Old El Paso	Wholewheat Tortillas	1.3 %
	Stand 'n' Stuff Soft Flour Tortillas	1.9 %
	Large Flour Tortillas	2.0 %
	Regular Flour Tortillas	2.5 %
	Mini Flour Tortillas	2.8 %
Pacificio Italiano	Olive Ciabatta	0.8 %

Breads - by brand (continued)

Brand	Label	% Sugar
Pacificio Italiano	Half Ciabatta	1.1 %
	Plain Ciabatta	1.1 %
Patak's	Plain Chapattis	2.5 %
	Plain Naans	2.9 %
	Garlic & Coriander Naans	3.0 %
Robert's Bakery	White Rolls	2.0 %
	White Danish Loaf	2.2 %
	White Farmhouse Loaf	2.2 %
	Thick White Loaf	2.3 %
	White Sourdough	2.3 %
	Wholemeal Loaf	2.3 %
	Floury Rolls	2.4 %
	50 % White 50 % Wholemeal Loaf	2.5 %
	Tiger Bloomer	2.6 %
	White Finger Rolls	2.6 %
	Seeded Farmhouse	2.7 %
	Soft White Deli Rolls	2.8 %
	Soft Brown Loaf	2.9 %
Sainsbury's	Be Good Plain Mini Naan	1.4 %
	Taste the Difference Garlic & Coriander Naan Bread	1.5 %
	Flamebaked Chapatti	1.6 %
	Flamebaked Garlic & Coriander Naan	1.6 %
	Flamebaked Plain Naan	1.8 %
	Taste the Difference Crumpets	1.8 %
	Chapattis	2.0 %

Breads - by brand (continued)

Brand	Label	% Sugar
Sainsbury's	Soft Flour Tortillas	2.1 %
	Be Good Plain Wraps	2.2 %
	Chilli & Garlic Naan	2.2 %
	Garlic & Coriander Naans	2.3 %
	SO Organic Sunflower & Pumpkin Seed Bread	2.3 %
	Plain Tortilla Wraps	2.5 %
	Wholemeal Tortillas Wraps	2.5 %
	Panini Rolls	2.6 %
	Plain Naans	2.6 %
	SO Organic Seeded Wholemeal Rolls	2.7 %
	Basics White Pitta	2.8 %
	Taste the Difference Wholemeal Bloomers	2.8 %
	Flamebaked Garlic & Parsley Flatbread	2.9 %
	Oat Topped Wholemeal Deli Rolls	3.0 %
	SO Organic Multiseeded Wholemeal Bread	3.0 %
Santa Maria	Corn & Wheat Soft Tortillas	2.0 %
	Wholemeal Soft Tortillas	2.7 %
Shana	Original Paratha	2.7 %
	Garlic Paratha	3.0 %
Sharwood's	Garlic & Coriander Mini Naans	2.2 %
	Plain Chapattis	2.5 %
Tesco	Traditional Spanish Tortilla	0.5 %
	Six Grain Loaf	0.8 %
	Bakery Seeded Panini	1.2 %
	Bakery Three Cheese Bread	1.2 %

Breads – by brand (continued)

Brand	Label	% Sugar
Tesco	Bakery Cheese Topped Sub	1.3 %
	Kalamata Olive Bloomer	1.3 %
	Bakery Chunky Cheese Roll	1.5 %
	Bakery Tiger Roll	1.5 %
	Mediterranean Herb Pitta Squares	1.5 %
	White Pitta	1.5 %
	Bakery Sour Dough Bloomer	1.6 %
	Finest Garlic & Coriander Naan Bread	1.6 %
	Bakery Ploughmans Cob	1.8 %
	Finest Plain Naan Bread	1.8 %
	Reduced Fat Plain Naan	1.8 %
	Wholemeal Pitta Squares	1.8 %
	Stay Fresh White Bread	1.9 %
	Bakery Panini	2.0 %
	Everyday Value Plain Naan Breads	2.0 %
	White Pitta Squares	2.0 %
	Finest Ciabatta	2.2 %
	Panini Rolls	2.2 %
	Plain Tortilla Wraps	2.2 %
	Stay Fresh Wholemeal Bread	2.2 %
	Stonebaked Ciabatta	2.3 %
	70 Calorie Wholemeal Bread	2.4 %
	Bakery Ciabatta Roll	2.4 %
	Bakery Organic White Bloomer	2.5 %
	Takeaway Plain Mega Naan	2.5 %
	Wholemeal Pitta	2.5 %

Breads - by brand (continued)

Brand	Label	% Sugar
Tesco	Bakery Crusty White Roll	2.6 %
	Bakery Organic Brown Bloomer	2.6 %
	Cheese & Garlic Flatbread	2.6 %
	Light Choices Mini Naan Bread	2.6 %
	Mediterranean Herb Tortilla Wraps	2.6 %
	Toastie White Bread	2.6 %
	Bakery Cheese Topped Roll	2.7 %
	Finest Stone Ground Wholemeal Farmhouse Bread	2.7 %
	Bakery Sesame Roll	2.8 %
	Bakery Soft Sub	2.8 %
	Everyday Value White Pitta Bread	2.8 %
	Finest Cornish All Butter Toasting Muffins	2.8 %
	Seeded Burger Buns	2.8 %
	Seeded Tortilla Wraps	2.8 %
	Bakery Salt & Pepper Bloomer	2.9 %
	Bakery Tiger Cheese Bloomer	2.9 %
	Plain Naan	2.9 %
	Bakery Cheese Topped Baton	3.0 %
	Bakery Corn Bread	3.0 %
	Bakery Poppy Seed Bloomer	3.0 %
	Bakery Rye Bread	3.0 %
	Everyday Value Crumpets	3.0 %
	Wholemeal Farmhouse Bread	3.0 %
The Food Doctor	Multi Seed & Cereal Pittas	2.0 %
	Multi Seed & Cereal Loaf	2.3 %

Breads – by brand (continued)

Brand	Label	% Sugar
The Polish Bakery	Rye 100 %	0.0 %
	Dark Rye Bread with Inulin	1.0 %
	Half Rye Half Wheat Bread	1.2 %
	Polish Style Caraway Seed Bread	1.2 %
	Poppy Seed Bread	1.2 %
	Brown Bread	1.5 %
	Sunflower Seed Bread	1.5 %
	Granny's Sesame Seed Bread	1.6 %
Udi's	White Sandwich Bread	1.1 %
	Brown Sandwich Bread	2.4 %
	Tiger Bloomer	2.6 %
	Classic Finger Rolls	2.7 %
Vogels	Sunflower & Barley	2.9 %
Waitrose	Stonebaked Ficelle Bread	0.5 %
	Essential Cheese & Garlic Tear & Share Bread	1.0 %
	Stonebaked Spelt Bread	1.0 %
	White Baguette	1.0 %
	Petit Pain	1.1 %
	Grand Rustic Bread	1.2 %
	Pain Rustica Bread	1.2 %
	Love Life Stoneground Wholemeal Loaf	1.4 %
	Roasted Garlic Ciabatta	1.6 %
	Farmhouse Wholemeal Loaf	1.7 %
	Love Life Gluten Free Seeded Loaf	1.7 %
	Wholemeal Long Tin Loaf	1.7 %

Breads – by brand (continued)

Brand	Label	% Sugar
Waitrose	Organic Brown Loaf	1.8 %
	Love Life Wholemeal & Seeds Bread	1.9 %
	Mixed Seeds Baguette	1.9 %
	Six Seeded Brown Batch Bread	2.0 %
	Heyford Wholemeal Bread	2.1 %
	Love Life Gluten Free White Pitta	2.1 %
	Stonebaked Boule	2.1 %
	Stonebaked Baguette	2.2 %
	Essential Plain Tortilla Wraps	2.3 %
	Essential Wholemeal Tortillas Wraps	2.3 %
	Paysan Rustica Bread	2.3 %
	Roasted Garlic Flatbread	2.3 %
	Essential Garlic Baguette	2.4 %
	White Flute Bread	2.4 %
	Essential Picnic White Pitta	2.5 %
	Grand Mange Paysan	2.5 %
	Mixed Olive Ficelle Bread	2.5 %
	Sourdough with Seeds Baguette	2.5 %
	Grand Mange Blanc	2.6 %
	Poppy Seed Roll	2.6 %
	Organic Farmhouse Wholegrain Loaf	2.7 %
	Indian Plain Parathas	2.8 %
	Love Life Farmhouse Batch Wholemeal Loaf	2.8 %
	Pain au Levain	2.8 %
	White with Wholemeal Loaf	2.8 %

Breads – by brand (continued)

Brand	Label	% Sugar
Waitrose	Essential Mini White Pitta	2.9 %
	Love Life Farmhouse Wholemeal & Pumpkin Loaf	3.0 %
	Love Life Wholemeal, Rye & Toasted Rye Grain Loaf	3.0 %
Warburtons	Soft House Farmhouse	1.7 %
	Thick & Fluffy Crumpets	2.0 %
	White Loaf	2.2 %
	Crusty White Loaf	2.3 %
	Danish White Loaf	2.3 %
	Sliced White Rolls	2.3 %
	Half & Half Loaf	2.4 %
	Wholemeal Loaf	2.4 %
	Old English White	2.6 %
	Seeded Batch Loaf	2.6 %
	Wholemeal Rolls	2.8 %
	Large White Rolls	2.9 %
	Tear & Toast Muffins	2.9 %
	White Sub Rolls	2.9 %
	Soft White Pitta Halves	3.0 %
Weight Watchers	Love Fibre Wraps	1.4 %
	Petit Pains	1.5 %
	Soft Brown Danish	2.2 %
	Garlic & Coriander Mini Naans	2.3 %
	Plain Mini Naans	2.4 %
	Soft Malted Danish	2.6 %

Breads - by brand (continued)

Brand	Label	% Sugar
Weight Watchers	Thick Sliced Wholemeal	2.6 %
	Garlic & Herb Ciabatta	2.7 %
	Garlic & Herb Petit Pains	2.7 %
	Soft White Danish	2.7 %

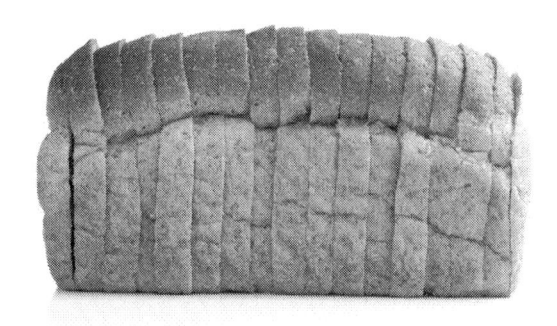

Biscuits

I've presented this list in two formats so you can browse by sugar content or brand. You might notice that all the biscuits in this list are essentially crackers. That's because the lowest sugar sweet biscuit you can get in Britain today is Sainsbury's Basics Shortbread Finger (12.8 percent sugar) and it's a long way outside the 3 percent rule.

Many of these biscuits will contain seed oils. If you are concerned about this, then use the fat reckoner chart available at www.howmuchsugar.com to determine whether your choice is likely to be as low in seed oil as it is in sugar.

Biscuits - by sugar content

Brand	Label	% Sugar
Arden's	Pesto Flavour Bakes	0.1 %
Clearspring	Extra Virgin Olive Oil Japanese Rice Crackers	0.1 %
Clearspring	Tamari Japanese Rice Crackers	0.1 %
Morrisons	Cheese Crispies	0.1 %
Amisa Organic	Gluten Free Amaranth Rice Crispbread	0.2 %
Clearspring	Organic Corn Cakes	0.2 %
Kent & Fraser	Sussex Farmer's Biscuits	0.2 %
Sainsbury's	Taste the Difference Cheddar & Black Pepper Bites	0.2 %
Waitrose	Mini Breadsticks	0.2 %
Amisa Organic	Gluten Free Grissini Corn & Rice Sticks	0.3 %
Amisa Organic	Poppy Seed Chilli Spelt Snack Sticks	0.3 %
Rude Health	Mini Corn Thins	0.3 %
Sainsbury's	Taste the Difference Cheddar Cheese Bites	0.3 %

Biscuits - by sugar content (continued)

Brand	Label	% Sugar
Sainsbury's	Taste the Difference Cheddar Cheese Crispies	0.3 %
Wasa	Sourdough Rye Crispbread	0.3 %
ASDA	Chosen by you Cheese Crackers	0.4 %
ASDA	Chosen by you Slightly Salted Rice Cakes	0.4 %
ASDA	Good & Counted Salt & Vinegar Rice Cakes	0.4 %
Kallo	Buckwheat Superseeds Multigrain Cakes	0.4 %
Morrisons	Lightly Salted Rice Cakes	0.4 %
Morrisons	Rough Scottish Oatcakes	0.4 %
Morrisons	Salt & Vinegar Rice Cakes	0.4 %
Real Foods	Organic Sesame Corn Thins	0.4 %
Rude Health	Corn Thins	0.4 %
Sainsbury's	Be Good Rice Cakes	0.4 %
Sakata	Lightly Salted Rice Crackers	0.4 %
Amisa Organic	Gluten Free Rice & Corn Crispbread	0.5 %
Biona Organic	No Salt Corn Cakes	0.5 %
Kallo	Lightly Salted Rice Cakes	0.5 %
Kallo	Organic Lightly Salted Corn Cake Thins	0.5 %
Kallo	Organic Lightly Salted Rice Cakes	0.5 %
Kallo	Organic Sesame Seed Rice Cakes	0.5 %
Kallo	Organic Unsalted Rice Cakes	0.5 %
Nature's Store	Natural Corn Cakes	0.5 %
Nature's Store	Quinoa Corn Cakes	0.5 %
Wasa	Sourdough Multigrain Crispbread	0.5 %
Le Veneziane	Mini Grissini Breadsticks	0.6 %
Nairn's	Cheese Oatcakes	0.6 %

Biscuits - by sugar content (continued)

Brand	Label	% Sugar
Nairn's	Organic Oatcakes	0.6 %
Organ	Essential Fibre Crispbread	0.6 %
Rude Health	Mini Rice Thins	0.6 %
Rude Health	Multigrain Thins	0.6 %
Sainsbury's	Taste the Difference Sea Salt & Black Pepper Crackers	0.6 %
Weight Watchers	Love Fibre Multigrain Rice Cakes	0.6 %
Biona Organic	Amaranth Rice Cakes	0.7 %
Crosta & Mollica	Fennel Seed Tarallini	0.7 %
DS Gluten Free	Rice Cakes	0.7 %
Nairn's	Cracked Black Pepper Oatcakes	0.7 %
Nature's Store	Slightly Salted Rice Cakes	0.7 %
Raw Health	Tomato Tarallini	0.7 %
Real Foods	Multigrain Corn Thins	0.7 %
Rude Health	Oat & Spelt Thins	0.7 %
Tesco	Scottish Rough Oatcakes	0.7 %
Waitrose	Love Life Fine Oatcakes	0.7 %
Amisa Organic	Gluten Free Veggie Garden Crispbread	0.8 %
Biona Organic	No Salt Rice Cakes	0.8 %
Biona Organic	Sea Salt Rice Cakes	0.8 %
Clearspring	Black Sesame Japanese Brown Rice Crackers	0.8 %
Clearspring	Sea Vegetable & Black Pepper Organic Oatcakes	0.8 %
Clearspring	Whole Sesame Japanese Brown Rice Crackers	0.8 %
Kallo	Spelt, Oat & Oat Bran Rice Cakes	0.8 %

Biscuits - by sugar content (continued)

Brand	Label	% Sugar
Marmite	Rice Cakes	0.8 %
Nairn's	Sunflower & Pumpkin Seed Oatcakes	0.8 %
Rakusen's	Cheese Matzo Snackers	0.8 %
Real Foods	Soy, Linseed & Chia Corn Thins	0.8 %
Rude Health	Brown Rice Thins	0.8 %
Sainsbury's	Rough Oatcakes	0.8 %
Tesco	Finest All Butter Cheese Straws	0.8 %
Arden's	Goats Cheese & Black Pepper Bites	0.9 %
ASDA	Chosen by you Original Scottish Oatcakes	0.9 %
Biona Organic	Quinoa Rice Cakes	0.9 %
Clearspring	Traditional Organic Oatcakes	0.9 %
Morrisons	Signature All Butter Pastry Pesto Hearts	0.9 %
Nairn's	Fine Milled Oatcakes	0.9 %
Nairn's	Mini Oatcakes	0.9 %
Nairn's	Organic Herb & Pumpkin Seed Oatcakes	0.9 %
Peckish	Sea Salt & Vinegar Rice Crackers	0.9 %
Peckish	Sour Cream & Chive Rice Crackers	0.9 %
Peckish	Tangy BBQ Rice Crackers	0.9 %
Real Foods	Wholegrain Rice Thins	0.9 %
Waitrose	Love Life Rough Oatcakes	0.9 %
Waitrose	Love Life Seeded Oatcakes	0.9 %
Crosta & Mollica	Chilli Crostini	1.0 %
Crosta & Mollica	Oregano Crostini	1.0 %
Jacob's	Cornish Wafers	1.0 %
Morrisons	Biscuits for Cheese	1.0 %
Roca	Pesto Cheese Crispies	1.0 %

Biscuits - by sugar content (continued)

Brand	Label	% Sugar
Sainsbury's	Corn Thins	1.0 %
Sainsbury's	Taste the Difference Black Onion Seed Crackers	1.0 %
Stockan's	Thin Oatcakes	1.0 %
Tesco	Biscuits for Cheese	1.0 %
Wasa	Falu Rag-rut Crispbread	1.0 %
Wasa	Original Crispbread	1.0 %
Wasa	Original Ricecakes	1.0 %
Wasa	Solrute Sesame Crispbread	1.0 %
ASDA	Chosen by you Cracked Black Pepper Scottish Oatcakes	1.1 %
Jacob's	Butter Puffs	1.1 %
Kallo	Savoury Rice Cakes	1.1 %
Roca	Cheese Crispies	1.1 %
Ryvita	Black Pepper Crackers	1.1 %
Ryvita	Golden Rye Crackers	1.1 %
Stoats	Chipotle Chilli Oatcakes	1.1 %
Arden's	Garlic & Parsley Swirls	1.2 %
Clearspring	Sundried Tomato & Herb Organic Oatcakes	1.2 %
Dr. Karg	Spelt & Cheese Crispbread	1.2 %
GG	Multi-Seed Crispbread	1.2 %
Kallo	Fairtrade Organic Sesame Seed Rice Cakes	1.2 %
Kallo	Fairtrade Organic Unsalted Rice Cakes	1.2 %
Peckish	Cheddar Cheese Rice Crackers	1.2 %
Sainsbury's	Butter Puffs	1.2 %

Biscuits - by sugar content (continued)

Brand	Label	% Sugar
Tesco	Finest Savoury Selection	1.2 %
Tesco	Lightly Salted Rice Cakes	1.2 %
Amisa Organic	Gluten Free Buckwheat Crispbread	1.3 %
Amisa Organic	Gluten Free Quinoa Fibre Crispbread	1.3 %
Clearspring	Sea Vegetable Japanese Rice Crackers	1.3 %
Dr. Karg	Seeded Spelt Crispbread	1.3 %
Finn Crisp	Crisp Garlic Thins	1.3 %
Nairn's	Rough Oatcakes	1.3 %
Stoats	Rustic Scottish Oatcakes	1.3 %
Thomas J. Fudges	Mature Cheddar Puffed Straws	1.3 %
ASDA	Chosen by you Cracker Selection	1.4 %
ASDA	Chosen by you Cream Crackers	1.4 %
Dr. Karg	3 Grains & 3 Seeds	1.4 %
Jacob's	Black Pepper Cream Crackers	1.4 %
Jacob's	Cream Crackers	1.4 %
Jacob's	Savours Salt & Cracked Black Pepper Bakes	1.4 %
Rakusen's	Traditional Matzos	1.4 %
Sainsbury's	Biscuits for Cheese Selection	1.4 %
Sainsbury's	Cream Crackers	1.4 %
Tesco	Cream Crackers	1.4 %
Waitrose	All Butter Cheddar Nibbles	1.4 %
Waitrose	Essential Cream Cackers	1.4 %
Carr's	Garlic & Herbs Table Water Biscuits	1.5 %
Carr's	Sesame Seeds Table Water Biscuits	1.5 %
Finn Crisp	Multigrain Thins	1.5 %

Biscuits - by sugar content (continued)

Brand	Label	% Sugar
Miller's Damsels	Wheat Wafers	1.5 %
Ryvita	Original Crackerbread	1.5 %
Sainsbury's	Parmesan & Basil Flatbread	1.5 %
Tesco	BBQ Rice Cakes	1.5 %
Thomas J. Fudges	Crispy Layered Cheddar & Chive Puffed Straws	1.5 %
Waitrose	Grissini Breadsticks	1.5 %
Wasa	Delikatess Lineseed	1.5 %
Wasa	Family Crisp Crispbread	1.5 %
Wasa	Husman Crispbread	1.5 %
Wasa	Sport Crispbread	1.5 %
ASDA	Extra Special Rustic Cracker Collection	1.6 %
Carr's	Black Pepper Table Water Biscuits	1.6 %
Carr's	Table Water Biscuits	1.6 %
Crosta & Mollica	Classic Bruschettine	1.6 %
Finn Crisp	Caraway-Kummin Thins	1.6 %
Finn Crisp	Organic Thins	1.6 %
Finn Crisp	Original Thins	1.6 %
Jacob's	Cheeselets	1.6 %
Jacob's	High Fibre Cream Crackers	1.6 %
Newburn Bakehouse	Sweet Chilli Cracker Thins	1.6 %
Robert's Bakery	Sandwich Thins	1.6 %
Ryvita	Cheese Crackerbread	1.6 %
Sainsbury's	Be Good Cream Crackers	1.6 %
Snack a Jacks	Salt & Vinegar Jumbo Rice Cakes	1.6 %

Biscuits - by sugar content (continued)

Brand	Label	% Sugar
Amisa Organic	Gluten Free Paprika & Chilli Crackers	1.7 %
ASDA	Good & Counted Original Rye Crispbread	1.7 %
Barkat	Gluten Free Matzo Crackers	1.7 %
Crosta & Mollica	Classic Torinesi Breadsticks	1.7 %
Crosta & Mollica	Parmesan & Poppy Seed Torinesi Breadsticks	1.7 %
Finn Crisp	Sesame & Fibre Thins	1.7 %
Morrisons	Dark Rye Crispbreads	1.7 %
Newburn Bakehouse	Blue Cheese Cracker Thins	1.7 %
Rakusen's	99 % Baked Wheat Crackers	1.7 %
Annabel Kermel	Cheesy Bread Sticks	1.8 %
ASDA	Chosen by you Water Biscuits	1.8 %
Dr. Karg	Emmental Cheese & Pumpkin Seed Crispbread	1.8 %
Organico	Classic Croccantini Crackers	1.8 %
Organico	Rosemary Croccantini Crackers	1.8 %
Organico	Spelt Grissini Breadsticks	1.8 %
Organico	Torinesi Grissini Breadsticks	1.8 %
Ryvita	Thins Bites Cheddar & Cracked Black Pepper Flatbreads	1.8 %
Sainsbury's	High Bake Water Biscuits	1.8 %
Snack a Jacks	Salt & Vinegar Rice Cakes	1.8 %
Tesco	Garlic Crackers	1.8 %
Tesco	High Baked Water Biscuits	1.8 %
Tesco	Sesame Breadsticks	1.8 %
Waitrose	Essential High Bake Water Biscuits	1.8 %

Biscuits – by sugar content (continued)

Brand	Label	% Sugar
Amisa Organic	Chia & Flax Spelt Crispbread	1.9 %
Kallo	Torinesi with Parmesan Breadsticks	1.9 %
Rakusen's	Tea Matzos	1.9 %
Ryvita	Pepper Crackerbread	1.9 %
Sainsbury's	Taste the Difference 5 Seed Flatbread	1.9 %
Sainsbury's	Taste the Difference Savoury Biscuit Selection	1.9 %
Allos	Amaranth Crispbread	2.0 %
Amisa Organic	Gluten Free Sesame & Onion Crackers	2.0 %
ASDA	Chosen by you Free From Gluten Crackerbreads	2.0 %
ASDA	Good & Counted Sesame Seed Crispbread	2.0 %
DS Gluten Free	High Fibre Crackers	2.0 %
Kallo	Torinesi Breadsticks	2.0 %
Kallo	Torinesi with Sesame Seeds Breadsticks	2.0 %
Love More	Crackerbreads	2.0 %
Morrisons	Cheese Twists	2.0 %
Ryvita	Sesame Crispbread	2.0 %
Sainsbury's	Sunflower & Pumpkin Multiseed Flatbread	2.0 %
Tesco	Olive Grissini Rubata	2.0 %
Thomas J. Fudges	Crispy Layered Chilli & Sun-Dried Tomato Puffed Straws	2.0 %
Thomas J. Fudges	Seed & Oat Flats	2.0 %
Waitrose	Oat & Chive Biscuits for Cheese	2.0 %
Wasa	Crack & Taste Tomato & Chesse Crackers	2.0 %
Wasa	Delikatess Crispbread	2.0 %

Biscuits - by sugar content (continued)

Brand	Label	% Sugar
Wasa	Delikatess Sesame Crispbread	2.0 %
Wasa	Frukost Wholegrain Crispbread	2.0 %
Wasa	Havre Crispbread	2.0 %
Wasa	Mineral Plus Crispbread	2.0 %
Wasa	Sesame Crispbread	2.0 %
Wasa	Sport + Crispbread	2.0 %
Crosta & Mollica	Black Olive Grissini Breadsticks	2.1 %
Eskal	Original Deli Crackers	2.1 %
Miller's Harvest	Three-Seed Crackers	2.1 %
No-No	Houmous Flatbreads	2.1 %
Sainsbury's	Poppy & Sesame Seed Thins	2.1 %
Waitrose	Sesame Grissini Breadsticks	2.1 %
Amisa Organic	Sesame & Black Cumin Spelt Snack Sticks	2.2 %
ASDA	Good & Counted Multigrain Crispbread	2.2 %
Crosta & Mollica	Classic Grissini Breadsticks	2.2 %
Fortt's	Original Bath Oliver Biscuits	2.2 %
Granforno	Sesame Grissini Breadsticks	2.2 %
Tesco	Multiseed Flatbreads	2.2 %
Tesco	Salt & Vinegar Rice Cakes	2.2 %
Weight Watchers	Love Fibre Original Oatcakes	2.2 %
Amisa Organic	Spelt Melba Toast	2.3 %
Doria	Doriano Crackers	2.3 %
Kent & Fraser	Stilton & Walnut Savoury Biscuits	2.3 %
Morrisons	Poppy & Sesame Seed Thins	2.3 %
Nairn's	Oat Crackers	2.3 %
Weight Watchers	Herb & Onion Oat & Wheat Crackers	2.3 %

Biscuits - by sugar content (continued)

Brand	Label	% Sugar
Amisa Organic	Onion & Linseed Spelt Crispbread	2.4 %
ASDA	Chosen by you Sesame Breadsticks	2.4 %
ASDA	Extra Special Green Olive Twists	2.4 %
Finn Crisp	Hi-Fibre Crispbread	2.4 %
Ryvita	Mediterranean Herbs Crispbread	2.4 %
Ryvita	Thins Cheddar & Cracked Black Pepper Flatbreads	2.4 %
Thomas J. Fudges	Multi Seed & Oat Crackers	2.4 %
Biona Organic	No Salt Spelt Cakes	2.5 %
Rakusen's	99 % Herb & Onion Crackers	2.5 %
Ryvita	Cracked Black Pepper Crispbread	2.5 %
Sainsbury's	Melba Toasts	2.5 %
Tesco	Finest All Butter Mature Cheese Oat Nibbles	2.5 %
Wasa	Falu Rag-rut Grov Crispbread	2.5 %
Wasa	Fibre Crispbread	2.5 %
Wasa	Glutenfritt Crispbread	2.5 %
Weight Watchers	Oat & Wheat Crackers	2.5 %
Amisa Organic	Gluten Free Multi Seed Crispbread	2.6 %
Crosta & Mollica	Carta Da Musica Crispbread	2.6 %
Finn Crisp	Multigrain Crispbread	2.6 %
Jacob's	Krackawheat	2.6 %
Jacob's	Multigrain Flatbreads	2.6 %
Morrisons	Water Biscuits	2.6 %
No-No	Guacamole Flatbreads	2.6 %
Ryvita	Sunflower Seeds & Oats Crispbread	2.6 %
Tesco	Finest Hint of Tomato & Chilli Oatcakes	2.6 %

Biscuits - by sugar content (continued)

Brand	Label	% Sugar
Thomas J. Fudges	Deep Black Charcoal Heart Cheese Biscuits	2.6 %
DS Gluten Free	Breadsticks	2.7 %
Finn Crisp	5 Wholegrains Crispbread	2.7 %
Finn Crisp	Original Rye Crispbread	2.7 %
Finn Crisp	Traditional Crispbread	2.7 %
Peppa Pig	Baked Cheese Bread Sticks	2.7 %
Sainsbury's	Highland Oatcakes	2.7 %
Sakata	Roast Tomato & Balsamic Rice Crackers	2.7 %
Snack a Jacks	Sweet Chilli Rice Cakes	2.7 %
Waitrose	Nigella Seed Biscuits for Cheese	2.7 %
Waitrose	Seeded Wheat Biscuits for Cheese	2.7 %
Blue Dragon	Cheese Flavour Rice Crackers	2.8 %
ASDA	Good & Counted Caramel Rice Cakes	2.8 %
Jacob's	Mixed Seed Flatbreads	2.8 %
Jacob's	Savours Sour Cream & Chives Thins	2.8 %
Morrisons	Wholegrain Melba Toasts	2.8 %
Rakusen's	Matzos	2.8 %
Sainsbury's	Grissini Breadsticks	2.8 %
Sakata	Sizzling BBQ Rice Crackers	2.8 %
Tesco	Italian Original Breadsticks	2.8 %
Tesco	Poppy & Sesame Thins	2.8 %
Waitrose	Essential Poppy & Sesame Seed Thins	2.8 %
ASDA	Chosen by you Breadsticks	2.9 %
ASDA	Chosen by you Salt & Pepper Crackers	2.9 %
ASDA	Extra Special Italian Black Olive Breadsticks	2.9 %

Biscuits – by sugar content (continued)

Brand	Label	% Sugar
Dr. Karg	Classic 3-Seed Crispbread	2.9 %
Kingsmill	White Sandwich Thins	2.9 %
Miller's Damsels	Charcoal Wafers	2.9 %
Morrisons	Sea Salt & Black Pepper Scalloped Crackers	2.9 %
Nature's Store	Gluten Free Cheese Crackers	2.9 %
Ryvita	Original Crispbread	2.9 %
Ryvita	Thins Multi-Seed Flatbreads	2.9 %
Sainsbury's	Salt & Pepper Crackers	2.9 %
Tesco	Original Mini Breadsticks	2.9 %
Arden's	Gruyere & Spinach Twists	3.0 %
Kallo	Sea Salt & Balsamic Rice Cakes	3.0 %
Raw Health	Deeply Dense Pitta Bread	3.0 %
Raw Health	Provencale Crispbread	3.0 %
Ryvita	Dark Rye Crispbread	3.0 %
Ryvita	Hint of Chilli Crispbread	3.0 %
Sainsbury's	Sesame Grissini Breadsticks	3.0 %
Sainsbury's	Taste the Difference Caramelised Onion Cheese Nibbles	3.0 %
Waitrose	All Butter Sundried Tomato Bites	3.0 %
Wasa	Crack & Taste Salted Crackers	3.0 %

Biscuits - by brand

Brand	Label	% Sugar
Allos	Amaranth Crispbread	2.0 %
Amisa Organic	Gluten Free Amaranth Rice Crispbread	0.2 %
	Gluten Free Grissini Corn & Rice Sticks	0.3 %
	Poppy Seed Chilli Spelt Snack Sticks	0.3 %
	Gluten Free Rice & Corn Crispbread	0.5 %
	Gluten Free Veggie Garden Crispbread	0.8 %
	Gluten Free Buckwheat Crispbread	1.3 %
	Gluten Free Quinoa Fibre Crispbread	1.3 %
	Gluten Free Paprika & Chilli Crackers	1.7 %
	Chia & Flax Spelt Crispbread	1.9 %
	Gluten Free Sesame & Onion Crackers	2.0 %
	Sesame & Black Cumin Spelt Snack Sticks	2.2 %
	Spelt Melba Toast	2.3 %
	Onion & Linseed Spelt Crispbread	2.4 %
	Gluten Free Multi Seed Crispbread	2.6 %
Annabel Kermel	Cheesy Bread Sticks	1.8 %
Arden's	Pesto Flavour Bakes	0.1 %
	Goats Cheese & Black Pepper Bites	0.9 %
	Garlic & Parsley Swirls	1.2 %
	Gruyere & Spinach Twists	3.0 %
ASDA	Chosen by you Cheese Crackers	0.4 %
	Chosen by you Slightly Salted Rice Cakes	0.4 %
	Good & Counted Salt & Vinegar Rice Cakes	0.4 %
	Chosen by you Original Scottish Oatcakes	0.9 %
	Chosen by you Cracked Black Pepper Scottish Oatcakes	1.1 %

Biscuits - by brand (continued)

Brand	Label	% Sugar
ASDA	Chosen by you Cracker Selection	1.4 %
	Chosen by you Cream Crackers	1.4 %
	Extra Special Rustic Cracker Collection	1.6 %
	Good & Counted Original Rye Crispbread	1.7 %
	Chosen by you Water Biscuits	1.8 %
	Chosen by you Free From Gluten Crackerbreads	2.0 %
	Good & Counted Sesame Seed Crispbread	2.0 %
	Good & Counted Multigrain Crispbread	2.2 %
	Chosen by you Sesame Breadsticks	2.4 %
	Extra Special Green Olive Twists	2.4 %
	Good & Counted Caramel Rice Cakes	2.8 %
	Chosen by you Breadsticks	2.9 %
	Chosen by you Salt & Pepper Crackers	2.9 %
	Extra Special Italian Black Olive Breadsticks	2.9 %
Barkat	Gluten Free Matzo Crackers	1.7 %
Biona Organic	No Salt Corn Cakes	0.5 %
	Amaranth Rice Cakes	0.7 %
	No Salt Rice Cakes	0.8 %
	Sea Salt Rice Cakes	0.8 %
	Quinoa Rice Cakes	0.9 %
	No Salt Spelt Cakes	2.5 %
Blue Dragon	Cheese Flavour Rice Crackers	2.8 %
Carr's	Garlic & Herbs Table Water Biscuits	1.5 %
	Sesame Seeds Table Water Biscuits	1.5 %
	Black Pepper Table Water Biscuits	1.6 %

Biscuits - by brand (continued)

Brand	Label	% Sugar
Carr's	Table Water Biscuits	1.6 %
Clearspring	Extra Virgin Olive Oil Japanese Rice Crackers	0.1 %
	Tamari Japanese Rice Crackers	0.1 %
	Organic Corn Cakes	0.2 %
	Black Sesame Japanese Brown Rice Crackers	0.8 %
	Sea Vegetable & Black Pepper Organic Oatcakes	0.8 %
	Whole Sesame Japanese Brown Rice Crackers	0.8 %
	Traditional Organic Oatcakes	0.9 %
	Sundried Tomato & Herb Organic Oatcakes	1.2 %
	Sea Vegetable Japanese Rice Crackers	1.3 %
Crosta & Mollica	Fennel Seed Tarallini	0.7 %
	Chilli Crostini	1.0 %
	Oregano Crostini	1.0 %
	Classic Bruschettine	1.6 %
	Classic Torinesi Breadsticks	1.7 %
	Parmesan & Poppy Seed Torinesi Breadsticks	1.7 %
	Black Olive Grissini Breadsticks	2.1 %
	Classic Grissini Breadsticks	2.2 %
	Carta Da Musica Crispbread	2.6 %
Doria	Doriano Crackers	2.3 %
Dr. Karg	Spelt & Cheese Crispbread	1.2 %
	Seeded Spelt Crispbread	1.3 %

Biscuits - by brand (continued)

Brand	Label	% Sugar
Dr. Karg	3 Grains & 3 Seeds	1.4 %
	Emmental Cheese & Pumpkin Seed Crispbread	1.8 %
	Classic 3-Seed Crispbread	2.9 %
DS Gluten Free	Rice Cakes	0.7 %
	High Fibre Crackers	2.0 %
	Breadsticks	2.7 %
Eskal	Original Deli Crackers	2.1 %
Finn Crisp	Crisp Garlic Thins	1.3 %
	Multigrain Thins	1.5 %
	Caraway-Kummin Thins	1.6 %
	Organic Thins	1.6 %
	Original Thins	1.6 %
	Sesame & Fibre Thins	1.7 %
	Hi-Fibre Crispbread	2.4 %
	Multigrain Crispbread	2.6 %
	5 Wholegrains Crispbread	2.7 %
	Original Rye Crispbread	2.7 %
	Traditional Crispbread	2.7 %
Fortt's	Original Bath Oliver Biscuits	2.2 %
GG	Multi-Seed Crispbread	1.2 %
Granforno	Sesame Grissini Breadsticks	2.2 %
Jacob's	Cornish Wafers	1.0 %
	Butter Puffs	1.1 %
	Black Pepper Cream Crackers	1.4 %
	Cream Crackers	1.4 %

Biscuits - by brand (continued)

Brand	Label	% Sugar
Jacob's	Savours Salt & Cracked Black Pepper Bakes	1.4 %
	Cheeselets	1.6 %
	High Fibre Cream Crackers	1.6 %
	Krackawheat	2.6 %
	Multigrain Flatbreads	2.6 %
	Mixed Seed Flatbreads	2.8 %
	Savours Sour Cream & Chives Thins	2.8 %
Kallo	Buckwheat Superseeds Multigrain Cakes	0.4 %
	Lightly Salted Rice Cakes	0.5 %
	Organic Lightly Salted Corn Cake Thins	0.5 %
	Organic Lightly Salted Rice Cakes	0.5 %
	Organic Sesame Seed Rice Cakes	0.5 %
	Organic Unsalted Rice Cakes	0.5 %
	Spelt, Oat & Oat Bran Rice Cakes	0.8 %
	Savoury Rice Cakes	1.1 %
	Fairtrade Organic Sesame Seed Rice Cakes	1.2 %
	Fairtrade Organic Unsalted Rice Cakes	1.2 %
	Torinesi with Parmesan Breadsticks	1.9 %
	Torinesi Breadsticks	2.0 %
	Torinesi with Sesame Seeds Breadsticks	2.0 %
	Sea Salt & Balsamic Rice Cakes	3.0 %
Kent & Fraser	Sussex Farmer's Biscuits	0.2 %
	Stilton & Walnut Savoury Biscuits	2.3 %
Kingsmill	White Sandwich Thins	2.9 %
Le Veneziane	Mini Grissini Breadsticks	0.6 %
Love More	Crackerbreads	2.0 %

Biscuits - by brand (continued)

Brand	Label	% Sugar
Marmite	Rice Cakes	0.8 %
Miller's Damsels	Wheat Wafers	1.5 %
	Charcoal Wafers	2.9 %
Miller's Harvest	Three-Seed Crackers	2.1 %
Morrisons	Cheese Crispies	0.1 %
	Lightly Salted Rice Cakes	0.4 %
	Rough Scottish Oatcakes	0.4 %
	Salt & Vinegar Rice Cakes	0.4 %
	Signature All Butter Pastry Pesto Hearts	0.9 %
	Biscuits for Cheese	1.0 %
	Dark Rye Crispbreads	1.7 %
	Cheese Twists	2.0 %
	Poppy & Sesame Seed Thins	2.3 %
	Water Biscuits	2.6 %
	Wholegrain Melba Toasts	2.8 %
	Sea Salt & Black Pepper Scalloped Crackers	2.9 %
Nairn's	Cheese Oatcakes	0.6 %
	Organic Oatcakes	0.6 %
	Cracked Black Pepper Oatcakes	0.7 %
	Sunflower & Pumpkin Seed Oatcakes	0.8 %
	Fine Milled Oatcakes	0.9 %
	Mini Oatcakes	0.9 %
	Organic Herb & Pumpkin Seed Oatcakes	0.9 %
	Rough Oatcakes	1.3 %
	Oat Crackers	2.3 %
Nature's Store	Natural Corn Cakes	0.5 %

Biscuits - by brand (continued)

Brand	Label	% Sugar
Nature's Store	Quinoa Corn Cakes	0.5 %
	Slightly Salted Rice Cakes	0.7 %
	Gluten Free Cheese Crackers	2.9 %
Newburn Bakehouse	Sweet Chilli Cracker Thins	1.6 %
	Blue Cheese Cracker Thins	1.7 %
No-No	Houmous Flatbreads	2.1 %
	Guacamole Flatbreads	2.6 %
Organ	Essential Fibre Crispbread	0.6 %
Organico	Classic Croccantini Crackers	1.8 %
	Rosemary Croccantini Crackers	1.8 %
	Spelt Grissini Breadsticks	1.8 %
	Torinesi Grissini Breadsticks	1.8 %
Peckish	Sea Salt & Vinegar Rice Crackers	0.9 %
	Sour Cream & Chive Rice Crackers	0.9 %
	Tangy BBQ Rice Crackers	0.9 %
	Cheddar Cheese Rice Crackers	1.2 %
Peppa Pig	Baked Cheese Bread Sticks	2.7 %
Rakusen's	Cheese Matzo Snackers	0.8 %
	Traditional Matzos	1.4 %
	99 % Baked Wheat Crackers	1.7 %
	Tea Matzos	1.9 %
	99 % Herb & Onion Crackers	2.5 %
	Matzos	2.8 %
Raw Health	Tomato Tarallini	0.7 %
	Deeply Dense Pitta Bread	3.0 %

Biscuits – by brand (continued)

Brand	Label	% Sugar
Raw Health	Provencale Crispbread	3.0 %
Real Foods	Organic Sesame Corn Thins	0.4 %
	Multigrain Corn Thins	0.7 %
	Soy, Linseed & Chia Corn Thins	0.8 %
	Wholegrain Rice Thins	0.9 %
Robert's Bakery	Sandwich Thins	1.6 %
Roca	Pesto Cheese Crispies	1.0 %
Roca	Cheese Crispies	1.1 %
Rude Health	Mini Corn Thins	0.3 %
	Corn Thins	0.4 %
	Mini Rice Thins	0.6 %
	Multigrain Thins	0.6 %
	Oat & Spelt Thins	0.7 %
	Brown Rice Thins	0.8 %
Ryvita	Black Pepper Crackers	1.1 %
	Golden Rye Crackers	1.1 %
	Original Crackerbread	1.5 %
	Cheese Crackerbread	1.6 %
	Thins Bites Cheddar & Cracked Black Pepper Flatbreads	1.8 %
	Pepper Crackerbread	1.9 %
	Sesame Crispbread	2.0 %
	Mediterranean Herbs Crispbread	2.4 %
	Thins Cheddar & Cracked Black Pepper Flatbreads	2.4 %
	Cracked Black Pepper Crispbread	2.5 %

Biscuits - by brand (continued)

Brand	Label	% Sugar
Ryvita	Sunflower Seeds & Oats Crispbread	2.6 %
	Original Crispbread	2.9 %
	Thins Multi-Seed Flatbreads	2.9 %
	Dark Rye Crispbread	3.0 %
	Hint of Chilli Crispbread	3.0 %
Sainsbury's	Taste the Difference Cheddar & Black Pepper Bites	0.2 %
	Taste the Difference Cheddar Cheese Bites	0.3 %
	Taste the Difference Cheddar Cheese Crispies	0.3 %
	Be Good Rice Cakes	0.4 %
	Taste the Difference Sea Salt & Black Pepper Crackers	0.6 %
	Rough Oatcakes	0.8 %
	Corn Thins	1.0 %
	Taste the Difference Black Onion Seed Crackers	1.0 %
	Butter Puffs	1.2 %
	Biscuits for Cheese Selection	1.4 %
	Cream Crackers	1.4 %
	Parmesan & Basil Flatbread	1.5 %
	Be Good Cream Crackers	1.6 %
	High Bake Water Biscuits	1.8 %
	Taste the Difference 5 Seed Flatbread	1.9 %
	Taste the Difference Savoury Biscuit Selection	1.9 %
	Sunflower & Pumpkin Multiseed Flatbread	2.0 %
	Poppy & Sesame Seed Thins	2.1 %

Biscuits - by brand (continued)

Brand	Label	% Sugar
Sainsbury's	Melba Toasts	2.5 %
	Highland Oatcakes	2.7 %
	Grissini Breadsticks	2.8 %
	Salt & Pepper Crackers	2.9 %
	Sesame Grissini Breadsticks	3.0 %
	Taste the Difference Caramelised Onion Cheese Nibbles	3.0 %
Sakata	Lightly Salted Rice Crackers	0.4 %
	Roast Tomato & Balsamic Rice Crackers	2.7 %
	Sizzling BBQ Rice Crackers	2.8 %
Snack a Jacks	Salt & Vinegar Jumbo Rice Cakes	1.6 %
	Salt & Vinegar Rice Cakes	1.8 %
	Sweet Chilli Rice Cakes	2.7 %
Stoats	Chipotle Chilli Oatcakes	1.1 %
	Rustic Scottish Oatcakes	1.3 %
Stockan's	Thin Oatcakes	1.0 %
Tesco	Scottish Rough Oatcakes	0.7 %
	Finest All Butter Cheese Straws	0.8 %
	Biscuits for Cheese	1.0 %
	Finest Savoury Selection	1.2 %
	Lightly Salted Rice Cakes	1.2 %
	Cream Crackers	1.4 %
	BBQ Rice Cakes	1.5 %
	Garlic Crackers	1.8 %
	High Baked Water Biscuits	1.8 %
	Sesame Breadsticks	1.8 %

Biscuits - by brand (continued)

Brand	Label	% Sugar
Tesco	Olive Grissini Rubata	2.0 %
	Multiseed Flatbreads	2.2 %
	Salt & Vinegar Rice Cakes	2.2 %
	Finest All Butter Mature Cheese Oat Nibbles	2.5 %
	Finest Hint of Tomato & Chilli Oatcakes	2.6 %
	Italian Original Breadsticks	2.8 %
	Poppy & Sesame Thins	2.8 %
	Original Mini Breadsticks	2.9 %
Thomas J. Fudges	Mature Cheddar Puffed Straws	1.3 %
	Crispy Layered Cheddar & Chive Puffed Straws	1.5 %
	Crispy Layered Chilli & Sun-Dried Tomato Puffed Straws	2.0 %
	Seed & Oat Flats	2.0 %
	Multi Seed & Oat Crackers	2.4 %
	Deep Black Charcoal Heart Cheese Biscuits	2.6 %
Waitrose	Mini Breadsticks	0.2 %
	Love Life Fine Oatcakes	0.7 %
	Love Life Rough Oatcakes	0.9 %
	Love Life Seeded Oatcakes	0.9 %
	All Butter Cheddar Nibbles	1.4 %
	Essential Cream Cackers	1.4 %
	Grissini Breadsticks	1.5 %
	Essential High Bake Water Biscuits	1.8 %
	Oat & Chive Biscuits for Cheese	2.0 %

Biscuits - by brand (continued)

Brand	Label	% Sugar
Waitrose	Sesame Grissini Breadsticks	2.1 %
	Nigella Seed Biscuits for Cheese	2.7 %
	Seeded Wheat Biscuits for Cheese	2.7 %
	Essential Poppy & Sesame Seed Thins	2.8 %
	All Butter Sundried Tomato Bites	3.0 %
Wasa	Sourdough Rye Crispbread	0.3 %
	Sourdough Multigrain Crispbread	0.5 %
	Falu Rag-rut Crispbread	1.0 %
	Original Crispbread	1.0 %
	Original Ricecakes	1.0 %
	Solrute Sesame Crispbread	1.0 %
	Delikatess Lineseed	1.5 %
	Family Crisp Crispbread	1.5 %
	Husman Crispbread	1.5 %
	Sport Crispbread	1.5 %
Wasa	Crack & Taste Tomato & Chesse Crackers	2.0 %
	Delikatess Crispbread	2.0 %
	Delikatess Sesame Crispbread	2.0 %
	Frukost Wholegrain Crispbread	2.0 %
	Havre Crispbread	2.0 %
	Mineral Plus Crispbread	2.0 %
	Sesame Crispbread	2.0 %
	Sport + Crispbread	2.0 %
	Falu Rag-rut Grov Crispbread	2.5 %
	Fibre Crispbread	2.5 %
	Glutenfritt Crispbread	2.5 %

Biscuits - by brand (continued)

Brand	Label	% Sugar
Wasa	Crack & Taste Salted Crackers	3.0 %
Weight Watchers	Love Fibre Multigrain Rice Cakes	0.6 %
	Love Fibre Original Oatcakes	2.2 %
	Herb & Onion Oat & Wheat Crackers	2.3 %
	Oat & Wheat Crackers	2.5 %

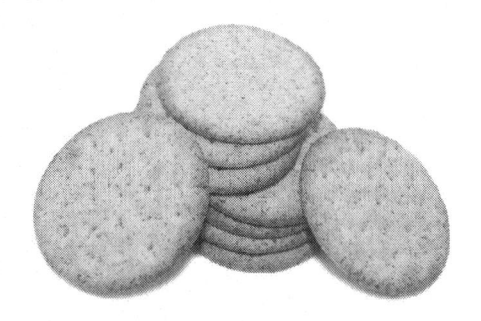

Frozen Pizza

I've presented this list in two formats so you can browse by sugar content or brand. The sugar contents have not been adjusted for any lactose in the cheese but that is not likely to be significant.

Most of these frozen pizzas will contain seed oils. If you are concerned about this, then use the fat reckoner chart available at www.howmuchsugar.com to determine whether your choice is likely to be as low in seed oil as it is in sugar.

Frozen Pizza - by sugar content

Brand	Label	% Sugar
Goodfella's	Cheesy Garlic Bread Pizza	0.8 %
ASDA	Cheese & Tomato Pizza	1.2 %
Chicago Town	The Deep Pan Triple Cheese Pizza	1.2 %
Waitrose	Crisp & Cheesy Cheese Feast Pizza	1.2 %
ASDA	Ham & Cheese Snack Pizza	1.3 %
Virtu	Mushroom Pizza Baguette	1.3 %
Waitrose	Crisp & Meaty Spicy Pepperoni Feast Pizza	1.3 %
Chicago Town	The Deep Dish Chicken Melt Pizza	1.5 %
Chicago Town	The Deep Dish Ham & Cheese Topper Pizza	1.5 %
ASDA	Pepperoni Pizza	1.6 %
Chicago Town	The Deep Dish Four Cheese Pizza	1.6 %
Chicago Town	The Deep Dish Pepperoni Pizza	1.6 %
Chicago Town	The Deep Pan Double Pepperoni Pizza	1.6 %
Sainsbury's	Taste the Difference Ham Hock, Red Onion & Goats' Cheese Pizza	1.6 %
Chicago Town	The Deep Dish Meat Combo Pizza	1.7 %
DS Gluten Free	Bonta d' Italia Margherita	1.7 %
DS Gluten Free	Bonta d' Italia Salami	1.7 %

Frozen Pizza - by sugar content (continued)

Brand	Label	% Sugar
Sainsbury's	Deep & Loaded Chilli Beef Pizza	1.7 %
Dr. Oetkar	Ristorante Funghi Pizza	1.8 %
Morrisons	Signature Smoked Ham, Mushroom & Mascarpone Pizza	1.8 %
Waitrose	Menu From Waitrose Buffalo Mozzarella & Tomato 10" Pizza	1.8 %
Waitrose	Thin & Crispy Spinach & Goats Cheese Pizza	1.8 %
Waitrose	Thin & Hand Stretched Four Seasons Pizza	1.8 %
Toscana	Salami and Chilli Pizza	1.9 %
Waitrose	Thin & Hand Stretched Ham & Mushroom Pizza	1.9 %
ASDA	Meat Feast Stuffed Crust Pizza	2.0 %
Dr. Oetkar	Ristorante Spinaci Pizza	2.0 %
Morrisons	Thin & Crispy Cheese & Tomato Pizza	2.0 %
Tesco	Big Night In The Big Cheese Pizza	2.0 %
ASDA	Free From Gluten Pepperoni Pizza	2.1 %
Chicago Town	The Takeaway Chicken & Bacon Melt Classic Crust Pizza	2.1 %
Dr. Oetkar	Ristorante Mozzarella Pizza	2.1 %
Morrisons	Thin & Crispy Pepperoni Pizza	2.1 %
Virtu	Ham Pizza Baguette	2.1 %
Waitrose	Essential Pepperoni Pizza	2.1 %
Chicago Town	The Takeaway Four Cheese Classic Crust Pizza	2.2 %
Sainsbury's	Deep & Loaded Cheese Feast Pizza	2.2 %
Sainsbury's	Taste the Difference Chicken & Chorizo Pizza	2.2 %
Sainsbury's	Thin & Crispy Pepperoni Pizza	2.2 %
Amy's Kitchen	Cheese Pizza	2.3 %

Frozen Pizza - by sugar content (continued)

Brand	Label	% Sugar
ASDA	Ham & Cheese Pizza	2.3 %
ASDA	Smartprice Cheese & Tomato Pizza	2.3 %
Chicago Town	The Deep Dish Ham & Pineapple Pizza	2.3 %
Sainsbury's	Deep & Loaded Pepperoni Pizza	2.3 %
Sainsbury's	Thin & Crispy Margherita Pizza	2.3 %
Sainsbury's	Thin & Crispy Pepperoni 10" Pizza	2.3 %
Tesco	Free From Gluten Cheese & Tomato Pizza	2.3 %
Waitrose	Essential Cheese & Tomato Pizza	2.3 %
Waitrose	Thin & Hand Stretched Mushroom, Bacon & Mascarpone Pizza	2.3 %
Waitrose	Thin & Hand Stretched Spicy Pepperoni Pizza	2.3 %
Amy's Kitchen	Margherita Pizza	2.4 %
ASDA	Cheese & Tomato Snack Pizza	2.4 %
ASDA	Stonebaked Mad 4 Cheese Pizza	2.4 %
Chicago Town	The Takeaway Pepperoni Plus Classic Crust Pizza	2.4 %
Curry Dave	Chicken Madras Indian Style Flatbread Pizza	2.4 %
Hungry Joe's	Hot Dog Pizza	2.4 %
Sainsbury's	Takeaway Meat Feast Pizza	2.4 %
Sainsbury's	Thin & Crispy Meat Feast 10" Pizza	2.4 %
Tesco	Italian Double Salami Pizza	2.4 %
Waitrose	Thin & Hand Stretched Pepperoni Pizza	2.4 %
ASDA	Thin & Crispy Stonebaked Double Pepperoni & Chorizo Pizza	2.5 %
Dr. Oetkar	Panebello Pomodor Mozzarella Deep Crust Pizza	2.5 %
Dr. Oetkar	Ristorante Pollo Pizza	2.5 %

Frozen Pizza - by sugar content (continued)

Brand	Label	% Sugar
Dr. Oetkar	Tradizionale Prosciutto-Funghi Pizza	2.5 %
Goodfella's	Takeaway Fully Loaded Pepperoni Pizza	2.5 %
Gran Cucina	4 Organic Stonebaked Cheese & Tomato Pizza	2.5 %
Morrisons	Deep Pan Mega Four Cheese Pizza	2.5 %
Morrisons	Takeaway Stuffed Crust Pepperoni Pile Up Pizza	2.5 %
Sainsbury's	Taste the Difference Ham, Mushroom & Mascarpone Pizza	2.5 %
Tesco	Italian Cajun Chicken & Cherry Peppers Pizza	2.5 %
Toscana	Chargrilled Peppers and Asparagus Pizza	2.5 %
Waitrose	Menu From Waitrose Buffalo Mozzarella & Tomato 9" Pizza	2.5 %
Waitrose	Menu From Waitrose Spicy Calabrian Salami 9" Pizza	2.5 %
Waitrose	Thin & Crispy Milano Salami & Prosciutto Cotto Pizza	2.5 %
Waitrose	Thin & Hand Stretched Margherita Pizza	2.5 %
ASDA	Cheese Feast Stuffed Crust Pizza	2.6 %
ASDA	Stonebaked Pep-Me-Up Pizza	2.6 %
Chicago Town	The Takeaway Four Cheese Stuffed Crust Pizza	2.6 %
Dr. Oetkar	Ristorante Speciale Pizza	2.6 %
Dr. Oetkar	Tradizionale Salame Pizza	2.6 %
Goodfella's	Takeaway Fully The Big Cheese Pizza	2.6 %
Sainsbury's	Deep & Loaded Ham & Pineapple Pizza	2.6 %
Sainsbury's	Stonebaked Ham & Grilled Mushroom Pizza	2.6 %
Sainsbury's	Taste the Difference Etruscan Pepperoni Pizza	2.6 %

Frozen Pizza - by sugar content (continued)

Brand	Label	% Sugar
Sainsbury's	Taste the Difference Mozzarella & Sunblushed Tomato Pizza	2.6 %
Sainsbury's	Thin & Crispy Cheese & Tomato 10" Pizza	2.6 %
Waitrose	Menu From Waitrose Spicy Calabrian Salami 10" Pizza	2.6 %
Waitrose	Thin & Hand Stretched Spinach & Ricotta Pizza	2.6 %
ASDA	Deep Pan Meat Feast Pizza	2.7 %
ASDA	Quick Bite Cheese & Tomato Pizza Snack	2.7 %
ASDA	Stonebaked Fajita Chicken 10 inch Pizza	2.7 %
Chicago Town	The Takeaway Sloppy Joe Classic Crust Pizza	2.7 %
Dr. Oetkar	Panebello Pepperoni Speciale Deep Crust Pizza	2.7 %
Dr. Oetkar	Tradizionale Mozzarella Pizza	2.7 %
Morrisons	Deep Pan Cheese & Tomato Pizza	2.7 %
Morrisons	Deep Pan Pepperoni Pizza	2.7 %
Sainsbury's	Thin & Crispy Vegetable Pizza	2.7 %
Tesco	Finest Italian Meats Pizza	2.7 %
Tesco	Finest Rostello Ham Chestnut Mushroom And Mascarpone Pizza	2.7 %
Tesco	Finest Rostello Ham Spinach & Ricotta Pizza	2.7 %
ASDA	Margherita Sharing Pizza	2.8 %
ASDA	Stonebaked Veggie Chilli Cheezilla Pizza	2.8 %
ASDA	Thin Stonebaked Vegetable Feast Pizza	2.8 %
Chicago Town	The Takeaway Pepperoni Plus Stuffed Crust Pizza	2.8 %
Goodfella's	Takeaway Fully Flamin' Fajita Chicken Pizza	2.8 %
Goodfella's	Takeaway Fully Mighty Meat Feast Pizza	2.8 %

Frozen Pizza – by sugar content (continued)

Brand	Label	% Sugar
Hungry Joe's	Sizzlin' Hot Pepperoni Pizza	2.8 %
Morrisons	Loaded Deep Pan Mighty Meaty Pizza	2.8 %
Pizza alla pala	Prosciutto Cotto & Salami, Mozzarella Cheese Pizza	2.8 %
Tesco	Cheese Pizza Subs	2.8 %
Tesco	Thin & Tasty Cheese Feast Pizza	2.8 %
Waitrose	Essential Thin & Crispy Pepperoni Pizza	2.8 %
Waitrose	Thin & Hand Stretched Mushroom, Pepper & Courgette Pizza	2.8 %
ASDA	Deep Pan Chilli Beef Pizza	2.9 %
Chicago Town	The Takeaway BBQ Sizzler Stuffed Crust Pizza	2.9 %
Dr. Oetkar	Ristorante Pollo Arrabiata	2.9 %
Dr. Oetkar	Ristorante Quattro Formaggi Pizza	2.9 %
Hungry Joe's	BBQ Chicken & Bacon Pizza	2.9 %
Hungry Joe's	Doner Kebab Pizza	2.9 %
Pizza Express	American Hot Pepperoni & Hot Peppers Pizza	2.9 %
Pizza Express	Romana La Reine Pizza	2.9 %
Pizza Mia	Meat Feast	2.9 %
Tesco	Deep Pan Meat Feast Pizza	2.9 %
Waitrose	Menu From Waitrose Fire Roasted Vegetable & Pesto 10" Pizza	2.9 %
Amy's Kitchen	Spinach Pizza	3.0 %
ASDA	Deep Pan Chicken & Mushroom Pizza	3.0 %
ASDA	Extra Thin & Crispy Ham & Mushroom Pizza	3.0 %
ASDA	Louisiana Cajun Chicken Pizza	3.0 %
ASDA	Thin & Crispy Chicken & Sweetcorn Pizza	3.0 %
ASDA	Thin & Crispy Four Cheese Pizza	3.0 %

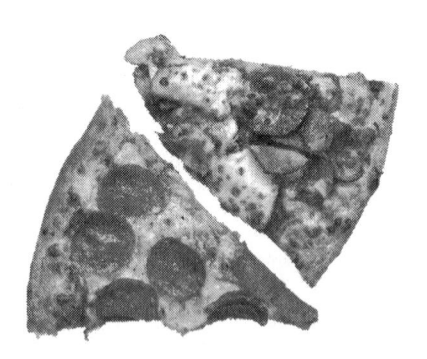

Frozen Pizza - by sugar content (continued)

Brand	Label	% Sugar
Curry Dave	Chicken Korma Indian Style Flatbread Pizza	3.0 %
Curry Dave	Chicken Tikka Masala Indian Style Flatbread Pizza	3.0 %
Goodfella's	Extra Thin Pepperoni & Chorizo Pizza	3.0 %
Morrisons	M Kitchen Deep Pan Spicy Chicken Pizza	3.0 %
Morrisons	M Kitchen Italian Cheese & Garlic Pizza Bread	3.0 %
Morrisons	Restaurant Style Margheritta Pizza	3.0 %
Pizza Express	Romana Giardineria Pizza	3.0 %
Pizza Mia	Pepperoni Pizza	3.0 %
Sainsbury's	Basics Cheese & Tomato Pizza	3.0 %
Sainsbury's	Stonebaked Mozzarella & Pesto Pizza	3.0 %
Waitrose	Essential Thin & Crispy British Ham, Mozzarella & Cheddar Pizza	3.0 %
Waitrose	Ultra Thin & Crispy Cherry Tomato, Asparagus & Pesto Pizza	3.0 %

Frozen Pizza - by brand

Brand	Label	% Sugar
Amy's Kitchen	Cheese Pizza	2.3 %
	Margherita Pizza	2.4 %
	Spinach Pizza	3.0 %
ASDA	Cheese & Tomato Pizza	1.2 %
	Ham & Cheese Snack Pizza	1.3 %
	Pepperoni Pizza	1.6 %
	Meat Feast Stuffed Crust Pizza	2.0 %
	Free From Gluten Pepperoni Pizza	2.1 %
	Ham & Cheese Pizza	2.3 %
	Smartprice Cheese & Tomato Pizza	2.3 %
	Cheese & Tomato Snack Pizza	2.4 %
	Stonebaked Mad 4 Cheese Pizza	2.4 %
	Thin & Crispy Stonebaked Double Pepperoni & Chorizo Pizza	2.5 %
	Cheese Feast Stuffed Crust Pizza	2.6 %
	Stonebaked Pep-Me-Up Pizza	2.6 %
	Deep Pan Meat Feast Pizza	2.7 %
	Quick Bite Cheese & Tomato Pizza Snack	2.7 %
	Stonebaked Fajita Chicken 10 inch Pizza	2.7 %
	Margherita Sharing Pizza	2.8 %
	Stonebaked Veggie Chilli Cheezilla Pizza	2.8 %
	Thin Stonebaked Vegetable Feast Pizza	2.8 %
	Deep Pan Chilli Beef Pizza	2.9 %
	Deep Pan Chicken & Mushroom Pizza	3.0 %
	Extra Thin & Crispy Ham & Mushroom Pizza	3.0 %
	Louisiana Cajun Chicken Pizza	3.0 %

Frozen Pizza - by brand (continued)

Brand	Label	% Sugar
ASDA	Thin & Crispy Chicken & Sweetcorn Pizza	3.0 %
	Thin & Crispy Four Cheese Pizza	3.0 %
Chicago Town	The Deep Pan Triple Cheese Pizza	1.2 %
	The Deep Dish Chicken Melt Pizza	1.5 %
	The Deep Dish Ham & Cheese Topper Pizza	1.5 %
	The Deep Dish Four Cheese Pizza	1.6 %
	The Deep Dish Pepperoni Pizza	1.6 %
	The Deep Pan Double Pepperoni Pizza	1.6 %
	The Deep Dish Meat Combo Pizza	1.7 %
	The Takeaway Chicken & Bacon Melt Classic Crust Pizza	2.1 %
	The Takeaway Four Cheese Classic Crust Pizza	2.2 %
	The Deep Dish Ham & Pineapple Pizza	2.3 %
	The Takeaway Pepperoni Plus Classic Crust Pizza	2.4 %
	The Takeaway Four Cheese Stuffed Crust Pizza	2.6 %
	The Takeaway Sloppy Joe Classic Crust Pizza	2.7 %
	The Takeaway Pepperoni Plus Stuffed Crust Pizza	2.8 %
	The Takeaway BBQ Sizzler Stuffed Crust Pizza	2.9 %
Curry Dave	Chicken Madras Indian Style Flatbread Pizza	2.4 %
	Chicken Korma Indian Style Flatbread Pizza	3.0 %
	Chicken Tikka Masala Indian Style Flatbread Pizza	3.0 %
Dr. Oetkar	Ristorante Funghi Pizza	1.8 %
	Ristorante Spinaci Pizza	2.0 %
	Ristorante Mozzarella Pizza	2.1 %
	Panebello Pomodor Mozzarella Deep Crust Pizza	2.5 %
	Ristorante Pollo Pizza	2.5 %

Frozen Pizza - by brand (continued)

Brand	Label	% Sugar
Dr. Oetkar	Tradizionale Prosciutto-Funghi Pizza	2.5 %
	Ristorante Speciale Pizza	2.6 %
	Tradizionale Salame Pizza	2.6 %
	Panebello Pepperoni Speciale Deep Crust Pizza	2.7 %
	Tradizionale Mozzarella Pizza	2.7 %
	Ristorante Pollo Arrabiata	2.9 %
	Ristorante Quattro Formaggi Pizza	2.9 %
DS Gluten Free	Bonta d' Italia Margherita	1.7 %
	Bonta d' Italia Salami	1.7 %
Goodfella's	Cheesy Garlic Bread Pizza	0.8 %
	Takeaway Fully Loaded Pepperoni Pizza	2.5 %
	Takeaway Fully The Big Cheese Pizza	2.6 %
	Takeaway Fully Flamin' Fajita Chicken Pizza	2.8 %
	Takeaway Fully Mighty Meat Feast Pizza	2.8 %
	Extra Thin Pepperoni & Chorizo Pizza	3.0 %
Gran Cucina	4 Organic Stonebaked Cheese & Tomato Pizza	2.5 %
Hungry Joe's	Hot Dog Pizza	2.4 %
	Sizzlin' Hot Pepperoni Pizza	2.8 %
	BBQ Chicken & Bacon Pizza	2.9 %
	Doner Kebab Pizza	2.9 %
Morrisons	Signature Smoked Ham, Mushroom & Mascarpone Pizza	1.8 %
	Thin & Crispy Cheese & Tomato Pizza	2.0 %
	Thin & Crispy Pepperoni Pizza	2.1 %
	Deep Pan Mega Four Cheese Pizza	2.5 %

Frozen Pizza - by brand (continued)

Brand	Label	% Sugar
Morrisons	Takeaway Stuffed Crust Pepperoni Pile Up Pizza	2.5 %
	Deep Pan Cheese & Tomato Pizza	2.7 %
	Deep Pan Pepperoni Pizza	2.7 %
	Loaded Deep Pan Mighty Meaty Pizza	2.8 %
	M Kitchen Deep Pan Spicy Chicken Pizza	3.0 %
	M Kitchen Italian Cheese & Garlic Pizza Bread	3.0 %
	Restaurant Style Margheritta Pizza	3.0 %
Pizza alla pala	Prosciutto Cotto & Salami, Mozzarella Cheese Pizza	2.8 %
Pizza Express	American Hot Pepperoni & Hot Peppers Pizza	2.9 %
	Romana La Reine Pizza	2.9 %
	Romana Giardineria Pizza	3.0 %
Pizza Mia	Meat Feast	2.9 %
	Pepperoni Pizza	3.0 %
Sainsbury's	Taste the Difference Ham Hock, Red Onion & Goats' Cheese Pizza	1.6 %
	Deep & Loaded Chilli Beef Pizza	1.7 %
	Deep & Loaded Cheese Feast Pizza	2.2 %
	Taste the Difference Chicken & Chorizo Pizza	2.2 %
	Thin & Crispy Pepperoni Pizza	2.2 %
	Deep & Loaded Pepperoni Pizza	2.3 %
	Thin & Crispy Margherita Pizza	2.3 %
	Thin & Crispy Pepperoni 10" Pizza	2.3 %
	Takeaway Meat Feast Pizza	2.4 %
	Thin & Crispy Meat Feast 10" Pizza	2.4 %
	Taste the Difference Ham, Mushroom & Mascarpone Pizza	2.5 %

Frozen Pizza – by brand (continued)

Brand	Label	% Sugar
Sainsbury's	Deep & Loaded Ham & Pineapple Pizza	2.6 %
	Stonebaked Ham & Grilled Mushroom Pizza	2.6 %
	Taste the Difference Etruscan Pepperoni Pizza	2.6 %
	Taste the Difference Mozzarella & Sunblushed Tomato Pizza	2.6 %
	Thin & Crispy Cheese & Tomato 10" Pizza	2.6 %
	Thin & Crispy Vegetable Pizza	2.7 %
	Basics Cheese & Tomato Pizza	3.0 %
	Stonebaked Mozzarella & Pesto Pizza	3.0 %
Tesco	Big Night In The Big Cheese Pizza	2.0 %
	Free From Gluten Cheese & Tomato Pizza	2.3 %
	Italian Double Salami Pizza	2.4 %
	Italian Cajun Chicken & Cherry Peppers Pizza	2.5 %
	Finest Italian Meats Pizza	2.7 %
	Finest Rostello Ham Chestnut Mushroom And Mascarpone Pizza	2.7 %
	Finest Rostello Ham Spinach & Ricotta Pizza	2.7 %
	Cheese Pizza Subs	2.8 %
	Thin & Tasty Cheese Feast Pizza	2.8 %
	Deep Pan Meat Feast Pizza	2.9 %
Toscana	Salami and Chilli Pizza	1.9 %
	Chargrilled Peppers and Asparagus Pizza	2.5 %
Virtu	Mushroom Pizza Baguette	1.3 %
	Ham Pizza Baguette	2.1 %
Waitrose	Crisp & Cheesy Cheese Feast Pizza	1.2 %
	Crisp & Meaty Spicy Pepperoni Feast Pizza	1.3 %

Frozen Pizza - by brand (continued)

Brand	Label	% Sugar
Waitrose	Menu From Waitrose Buffalo Mozzarella & Tomato 10" Pizza	1.8 %
	Thin & Crispy Spinach & Goats Cheese Pizza	1.8 %
	Thin & Hand Stretched Four Seasons Pizza	1.8 %
	Thin & Hand Stretched Ham & Mushroom Pizza	1.9 %
	Essential Pepperoni Pizza	2.1 %
	Essential Cheese & Tomato Pizza	2.3 %
	Thin & Hand Stretched Mushroom, Bacon & Mascarpone Pizza	2.3 %
	Thin & Hand Stretched Spicy Pepperoni Pizza	2.3 %
	Thin & Hand Stretched Pepperoni Pizza	2.4 %
	Menu From Waitrose Buffalo Mozzarella & Tomato 9" Pizza	2.5 %
	Menu From Waitrose Spicy Calabrian Salami 9" Pizza	2.5 %
	Thin & Crispy Milano Salami & Prosciutto Cotto Pizza	2.5 %
	Thin & Hand Stretched Margherita Pizza	2.5 %
	Menu From Waitrose Spicy Calabrian Salami 10" Pizza	2.6 %
	Thin & Hand Stretched Spinach & Ricotta Pizza	2.6 %
	Essential Thin & Crispy Pepperoni Pizza	2.8 %
	Thin & Hand Stretched Mushroom, Pepper & Courgette Pizza	2.8 %
	Menu From Waitrose Fire Roasted Vegetable & Pesto 10" Pizza	2.9 %
	Essential Thin & Crispy British Ham, Mozzarella & Cheddar Pizza	3.0 %
	Ultra Thin & Crispy Cherry Tomato, Asparagus & Pesto Pizza	3.0 %

Ready Meals

I've presented this list in two formats so you can browse by sugar content or brand.

Most of these ready meals will contain seed oils. If you are concerned about this, then use the fat reckoner chart available at www.howmuchsugar.com to determine whether your choice is likely to be as low in seed oil as it is in sugar.

Ready Meals - by sugar content

Brand	Label	% Sugar
Amy's Kitchen	Gluten Dairy Free Rice Mac & Cheeze	0.0 %
Morrisons	M Kitchen Chinese Takeaway Egg Fried Rice	0.0 %
ASDA	Chicken & Bacon Puff Pastry Lattice	0.1 %
ASDA	Chicken & Ham Bakes	0.1 %
ASDA	Classic Cottage Pie	0.1 %
ASDA	Classic Cumberland Pie	0.1 %
ASDA	Classic Fish Pie	0.1 %
ASDA	Classic Roast Beef Dinner in a Giant Yorkshire	0.1 %
ASDA	Classic Roast Chicken Dinner	0.1 %
ASDA	Extra Special Luxury Fish Pie	0.1 %
ASDA	Family Chicken & Vegetable Puff Pastry Pie	0.1 %
Morrisons	M Kitchen Tastes of Home Liver & Bacon with Mash	0.1 %
Morrisons	Steak & Ale Puff Pastry Pie	0.1 %
Mumtaz	Chicken Dopiaza & Pilau Rice	0.1 %
Pieminister	Moo Pie	0.1 %
Tesco	Everyday Value Chicken in White Sauce	0.1 %

Ready Meals - by sugar content (continued)

Brand	Label	% Sugar
Tesco	Finest Crab, Rocket & Chilli Linguine	0.1 %
Waitrose	Spaghetti Bolognese	0.1 %
ASDA	Classic Favourites Chicken Wrapped in Bacon	0.2 %
ASDA	Classic Favourites Ham & Mushroom Chicken	0.2 %
ASDA	Classic Gammon Dinner	0.2 %
ASDA	Classic Haddock & Chips	0.2 %
ASDA	Italian Chicken & Pesto Penne Pasta	0.2 %
ASDA	Steak & Kidney Puff Pastry Pie	0.2 %
ASDA	Tiger Cheese & Onion Puff Pastry Pie	0.2 %
Look What We Found!	Staffordshire Chicken Casserole	0.2 %
Morrisons	Savers Chicken in White Sauce	0.2 %
Mumtaz	Chicken Karahi & Pilau Rice	0.2 %
Pieminister	The Free Ranger Pie	0.2 %
Toscana	Mushroom Risotto	0.2 %
Waitrose	Mushroom Risotto	0.2 %
ASDA	Chicken Tikka Masala & Jalfrezi for 2	0.3 %
ASDA	Classic Favourites Chicken Kiev	0.3 %
ASDA	Classic Roast Beef Dinner	0.3 %
ASDA	Family Minced Steak & Onion Puff Pastry Pie	0.3 %
ASDA	Kids Chicken Tikka Masala	0.3 %
ASDA	Steak & Ale Puff Pastry Pie	0.3 %
Morrisons	M Kitchen Tastes of Home Sausage & Mash	0.3 %
Morrisons	Signature Coq Au Vin	0.3 %
Mumtaz	Chicken Korma & Pilau Rice	0.3 %
Tesco	Al Fresco Chicken & Chorizo Paella	0.3 %

Ready Meals – by sugar content (continued)

Brand	Label	% Sugar
Tesco	Finest King Prawn Spaghetti	0.3 %
Tesco	Finest Smoked Haddock Risotto	0.3 %
Tesco	Takeaway No 26 Vegetable Chow Mein	0.3 %
Waitrose	Menu Fish Pie	0.3 %
ASDA	Classic Chicken Breasts in Red Wine Sauce for 2	0.4 %
ASDA	Classic Favourites Cod Pie	0.4 %
ASDA	Classic Favourites Gammon & Cheese	0.4 %
ASDA	Classic Roast Pork Dinner with Crackling	0.4 %
ASDA	Family Steak & Potato Puff Pastry Pie	0.4 %
ASDA	Steak & Stilton Puff Pastry Pie	0.4 %
Charlie Bingham's	Chicken Kiev	0.4 %
Fray Bentos	Classic Steak & Kidney Pie	0.4 %
Fray Bentos	Deep Fill Just Steak Pie	0.4 %
Fray Bentos	Tender Just Steak Pie	0.4 %
Kirsty's	Thai Chilli Chicken with Rice Noodles	0.4 %
Morrisons	Savers Cottage Pie	0.4 %
Morrisons	Steak Puff Pastry Pie	0.4 %
Peter's	Steak & Kidney Pie	0.4 %
Princes	Italian Tuna Salad	0.4 %
Tesco	Everyday Value Chilled Cottage Pie	0.4 %
Waitrose	Beef Stroganoff	0.4 %
Waitrose	Chicken in Red Wine	0.4 %
Waitrose	Heston Slow-Cooked Pork	0.4 %
ASDA	Classic Favourites Cod with Cheese Sauce	0.5 %
ASDA	Classic Ham Hock in Parsley Sauce & Mash	0.5 %

Ready Meals - by sugar content (continued)

Brand	Label	% Sugar
ASDA	Good & Counted Chicken Enchiladas	0.5 %
ASDA	Spaghetti Bolognese	0.5 %
ASDA	World Favourites Lime & Coriander Chicken	0.5 %
Cook	Salmon & Dill Tart	0.5 %
Fray Bentos	Just Chicken Pies	0.5 %
Fray Bentos	Just Steak Pudding	0.5 %
Fray Bentos	Steak & Kidney Pudding	0.5 %
Kingston Town	Jerk Chicken with Rice & Peas	0.5 %
Morrisons	M Kitchen Italian Chicken Risotto	0.5 %
Morrisons	M Kitchen Tastes of Home Braised Beef & Mash	0.5 %
Morrisons	M Kitchen Tastes of Home Slow-Cooked Beef Brisket with Gravy	0.5 %
Morrisons	M Kitchen Tex Mex Southern Fried-Style Chicken with Curly Fries	0.5 %
Morrisons	Steak & Ale Large Puff Pastry Pie	0.5 %
Morrisons	Steak Large Shortcrust Pie	0.5 %
Mumtaz	Chicken Tikka Masala & Pilau Rice	0.5 %
Sainsbury's	Basics Cottage Pie	0.5 %
Sainsbury's	Chicken & Mushroom Casserole	0.5 %
Sainsbury's	Chicken in White Sauce	0.5 %
Sainsbury's	Classic Chicken Supreme	0.5 %
Tasty Favourites	Chicken & Mushrooms With Rice	0.5 %
Tesco	Chicken Curry	0.5 %
Tesco	Everyday Value Sausage And Mash	0.5 %
Tesco	Tex Mex Chicken Fajitas	0.5 %

Ready Meals - by sugar content (continued)

Brand	Label	% Sugar
Waitrose	Frozen Mini Cottage Pie	0.5 %
Waitrose	Love Life Fish Pie	0.5 %
Amy's Kitchen	Cheddar, Rice & Bean Burrito	0.6 %
ASDA	Chicken & Gravy Shortcrust Pastry Pie	0.6 %
ASDA	Classic Hunter's Chicken	0.6 %
ASDA	Classic Roast Chicken Dinner in a Giant Yorkshire	0.6 %
ASDA	Cottage Pie	0.6 %
ASDA	Indian Hot & Spicy Chicken Tikka Masala with Palau Rice & Bombay Potatoes	0.6 %
ASDA	Italian Chicken & Mushroom Risotto	0.6 %
ASDA	Kids Roast Chicken Dinner	0.6 %
ASDA	Steak & Gravy Puff Pastry Pie	0.6 %
ASDA	Steak & Gravy Shortcrust Pastry Pie	0.6 %
Birds Eye	Homebake Cheese & Onion Rolls	0.6 %
Bisto	Cottage Pie	0.6 %
Cook	Pork Dijon	0.6 %
Fray Bentos	Deep Fill Chicken & Mushroom Pie	0.6 %
Georgia's Choice	Chicken & Mushroom Crispy Bake	0.6 %
Morrisons	M Kitchen Tastes of Home Chicken & Mushroom Cumberland Pie	0.6 %
Morrisons	M Kitchen Tastes of Home Fisherman's Pie	0.6 %
Morrisons	Steak Small Puff Pastry Pie	0.6 %
Sainsbury's	Chicken & Mushroom Risotto	0.6 %
Tesco	Chicken in White Sauce	0.6 %
Tesco	Everyday Value Fisherman's Pie	0.6 %

Ready Meals - by sugar content (continued)

Brand	Label	% Sugar
Waitrose	Braised Beef and Mash	0.6 %
Waitrose	Fisherman's Pie	0.6 %
Waitrose	Heston Fish Pie	0.6 %
Waitrose	Menu Chicken Tarragon	0.6 %
Waitrose	Oriental Egg Fried Rice	0.6 %
Weight Watchers From Heinz	Chicken Curry	0.6 %
Young's	Chip Shop Fish Steak & Chips	0.6 %
Tesco	British Classics Fish Pie	0.7 %
Amoy	Malaysian Laksa Meal Kit	0.7 %
Amoy	Thai Red Curry Meal Kit	0.7 %
ASDA	Chicken & Gravy Large Puff Pastry Pie	0.7 %
ASDA	Chicken Shortcrust Pie	0.7 %
ASDA	Classic Chicken Bacon And Leek Pie for 2	0.7 %
ASDA	Family Favourites Cottage Pie	0.7 %
ASDA	Minced Steak & Onion Puff Pastry Pie	0.7 %
ASDA	Pork Sausage & Onion Puff Pastry Plait	0.7 %
ASDA	Steak & Gravy Large Shortcrust Pastry Pie	0.7 %
ASDA	Vegetarian Creamy Potato, Cheese & Onion Pie	0.7 %
Aunt Bessie's	Cheese & Onion Potato Bake	0.7 %
Charlie Bingham's	Breton Chicken	0.7 %
Charlie Bingham's	Chicken Wrapped in Prosciutto	0.7 %
Morrisons	Classic Fish & Chips	0.7 %
Morrisons	M Kitchen Fresh Ideas Mini Roast Chicken Dinner	0.7 %

Ready Meals – by sugar content (continued)

Brand	Label	% Sugar
Morrisons	M Kitchen Fresh Ideas Smoky Bacon Chicken	0.7 %
Morrisons	M Kitchen Italian Macaroni Cheese with Bacon	0.7 %
Morrisons	M Kitchen Tastes of Home Slow-Cooked Beef Rib in Gravy	0.7 %
Morrisons	Signature British Steak Diane	0.7 %
Morrisons	Signature Smoked Haddock & King Prawn Fish Pie	0.7 %
Morrisons	Steak & Kidney Small Shortcrust Pie	0.7 %
Our Little Secret	Delightful Carrot & Herb Rice	0.7 %
Peter's	Premier Steak Pie	0.7 %
Tesco	Finest Chicken Madeira and Braised Rice with Mushrooms	0.7 %
Tesco	Finest Spaghetti Carbonara	0.7 %
UpperCrust	Deep Filled Steak Pie	0.7 %
Waitrose	Heston Cauliflower Macaroni Cheese	0.7 %
Waitrose	Menu Mushroom Risotto	0.7 %
Weight Watchers	Chicken & Mushroom Pie	0.7 %
Young's	Fish Fillet Quarter Pounder & Chips	0.7 %
Young's	Gastro Cod Spinach, Cheese & Potato Gratin	0.7 %
Amoy	Thai Green Curry Meal Kit	0.8 %
ASDA	Bistro Ultimate Steak Pie	0.8 %
ASDA	Chicken & Mushroom with Egg Fried Rice	0.8 %
ASDA	Classic Favourites Peppercorn Chicken	0.8 %
ASDA	Classic Sausage & Mash	0.8 %
ASDA	Extra Special Salmon en Croute	0.8 %
ASDA	Family Size Deep Filled Chicken & Vegetable Pie	0.8 %

Ready Meals - by sugar content (continued)

Brand	Label	% Sugar
ASDA	Italian Chicken & Pesto Pasta Melt	0.8 %
ASDA	Italian Ham, Mushroom & Mascarpone Pasta Melt for 2	0.8 %
ASDA	Minced Beef & Onion Shortcrust Pie	0.8 %
ASDA	Prawn Curry & Rice	0.8 %
ASDA	Roast Chicken Dinner	0.8 %
ASDA	Smartprice Sausage and Mash	0.8 %
ASDA	Steak Pie	0.8 %
Bisto	Shepherd's Pie	0.8 %
Charlie Bingham's	Beef Stroganoff & Rice	0.8 %
Charlie Bingham's	Chicken en Croute	0.8 %
Charlie Bingham's	Steak & Ale Pies	0.8 %
Cook	Tarka Dal	0.8 %
Ginsters	Steak Pie	0.8 %
John West	Steam Pot Tuna with Chilli & Garlic and Spicy Red Pepper Couscous	0.8 %
Morrisons	M Kitchen Italian Ham & Mushroom Tagliatelle	0.8 %
Morrisons	NuMe Chicken Dinner	0.8 %
Princes	Chicken Casserole	0.8 %
Princes	Chicken in White Sauce	0.8 %
Pukka-Pies	Steak & Ale Pie	0.8 %
Sainsbury's	Pub Specials Chicken, Ham Hock & Leek Pies	0.8 %
Sharwood's	Chinese Chicken Rice	0.8 %
Smart-GF Kids	Brilliant Bolognese	0.8 %

Ready Meals - by sugar content (continued)

Brand	Label	% Sugar
Tesco	Al Fresco Polenta & Smoked Mozzarella	0.8 %
Tesco	Chicken Fajita Puff Pastry Pie	0.8 %
Tesco	Everyday Value Cheese Omelettes	0.8 %
Tesco	Finest Aberdeen Angus Cottage Pie	0.8 %
Tesco	Finest Beef Stroganoff with Wild Rice	0.8 %
Tesco	Finest Slow Cooked Steak Ragu with Pappardelle	0.8 %
Tesco	Healthy Living Chicken Chow Mein	0.8 %
Tesco	Italian Creamy Cheese & Bacon Spaghetti	0.8 %
Tesco	Takeaway Chinese Chicken Curry with Egg Fried Rice & Prawn Crackers	0.8 %
Tesco	British Classics Beef Roast Dinner	0.8 %
Tesco	British Classics Minced Lamb Hotpot	0.8 %
UpperCrust	Deep Filled Chicken & Asparagus Pie	0.8 %
Waitrose	Cottage Pie	0.8 %
Waitrose	Love Life Beef Fettuccine	0.8 %
Waitrose	Menu Chicken & Asparagus Risotto	0.8 %
Waitrose	Oriental Special Fried Rice	0.8 %
Weight Watchers From Heinz	Chicken & Lemon Risotto	0.8 %
Weight Watchers From Heinz	Chicken & Mushroom Tagliatelle	0.8 %
Young's	Scampi Bites & Chips	0.8 %
ASDA	Bistro Pork, Bramley Apple & Cider Pie	0.9 %
ASDA	Chicken & White Wine Puff Pastry Pie	0.9 %
ASDA	Chicken Tikka Masala with Pilau Rice	0.9 %

Ready Meals - by sugar content (continued)

Brand	Label	% Sugar
ASDA	Classic Chicken, Leek & Bacon Pie	0.9 %
ASDA	Extra Special King Prawn Linguine	0.9 %
ASDA	Extra Special Spiced Lamb with Bombay Potatoes & Tarka Dahl	0.9 %
ASDA	Indian Creamy Butter Chicken Masal with Pilau Rice & Bhajis	0.9 %
ASDA	Italian Spaghetti Carbonara	0.9 %
ASDA	Pub Classics Sausage & Mash	0.9 %
ASDA	Smartprice Fish Pie	0.9 %
ASDA	Steak & Ale Large Puff Pastry Pie	0.9 %
ASDA	Steak & Kidney Puff Pastry Pie	0.9 %
ASDA	Steak & Onion Puff Pastry Lattice	0.9 %
ASDA	Steak & Red Wine Large Puff Pastry Pie	0.9 %
Charlie Bingham's	Chicken Breasts with White Wine Sauce & Mash	0.9 %
Cook	Chicken Catalan	0.9 %
Cook	Chicken Pho	0.9 %
Cook	Classic Fish Pie	0.9 %
Fray Bentos	Deep Fill Steak & Ale Pie	0.9 %
Georgia's Choice	Fish Cakes	0.9 %
Higgidy	Little Mushroom, Feta & Spinach Pie	0.9 %
Little Dish	Fish Pie with Salmon and Pollock	0.9 %
Morrisons	Cumberland Pie	0.9 %
Morrisons	M Kitchen Tastes of Home Braised Steak & Mash	0.9 %
Morrisons	Signature British Rump Steak Stroganoff & Buttered Rice	0.9 %
Morrisons	Signature Cottage Pie with Real Ale Gravy	0.9 %

Ready Meals - by sugar content (continued)

Brand	Label	% Sugar
Morrisons	Signature King Prawn & Slow Roasted Tomato Linguine	0.9 %
Pukka-Pies	Large Potato and Meat Pie	0.9 %
Quorn	Meat Free Spaghetti Bolognese	0.9 %
Sainsbury's	Steak Family Pie	0.9 %
Tesco	Classic Italian Tuna Pasta Bake	0.9 %
Tesco	Everyday Value Cheese & Onion Quiche	0.9 %
Tesco	Family Favourites Mild Chilli con Carne with Rice	0.9 %
Tesco	Finest Cod & Crab Bake	0.9 %
Tesco	Finest Slow Cooked West Country Large Steak Pie	0.9 %
Toscana	Vegetable Risotto	0.9 %
Waitrose	Beef Goulash	0.9 %
Waitrose	Love Life Cottage Pie	0.9 %
Waitrose	Spaghetti Carbonara	0.9 %
Young's	Gastro Gratin Dauphinoise Fish Pie	0.9 %
Tesco	British Classics Beef Casserole & Dumplings	0.9 %
ASDA	Deep Filled Slow-Cooked Steak & Gravy Pie	1.0 %
ASDA	Extra Special Slow-Cooked Beef Stroganoff	1.0 %
ASDA	Extra Special West Country Beef Cottage Pie with Gentleman Jack Ale	1.0 %
ASDA	Kids Macaroni Cheese with Veg	1.0 %
ASDA	Peppered Steak Puff Pastry Pie	1.0 %
Bisto	Bangers & Mash	1.0 %
Charlie Bingham's	Beef Bourguignon & Potato Dauphinoise	1.0 %

Ready Meals - by sugar content (continued)

Brand	Label	% Sugar
Charlie Bingham's	Chicken & Mushroom Pies	1.0 %
Higgidy	Crustless Smoked English Bacon & Mature Cheddar Quiche	1.0 %
Morrisons	Chicken & Mushroom Puff Pastry Pie	1.0 %
Morrisons	Classic Steak Pie & Chips	1.0 %
Morrisons	M Kitchen Tastes of Home Beef Casserole	1.0 %
Morrisons	M Kitchen Tastes of Home Cottage Pie	1.0 %
Morrisons	Signature Wiltshire-Cured Ham & Chestnut Mushroom Tagliatelle	1.0 %
Pukka-Pies	Large Steak & Kidney Pie	1.0 %
Sainsbury's	Chicken & Gravy Family Pie	1.0 %
Sharwood's	Chicken Curry with Rice	1.0 %
Tesco	Classic Italian Macaroni Cheese	1.0 %
Tesco	Creamy Chicken & Bacon Puff Pastry Pie	1.0 %
Tesco	Finest Chicken with Italian Pancetta & Mozzarella	1.0 %
Tesco	Finest Roast Chicken & Gravy Pie	1.0 %
Tesco	Finest Shepherds Pie	1.0 %
Tesco	Slow Cooked Steak & Kidney Suet Pudding	1.0 %
Tesco	British Classics Large Cottage Pie	1.0 %
Tesco	British Classics Minced Beef & Mash	1.0 %
Tesco	British Classics Shepherd's Pie	1.0 %
Tesco	Egg Fried Rice	1.0 %
Tesco	Takeaway No 24 Egg Fried Rice	1.0 %
Uncle Ben's	Chicken & Mushroom Risotto	1.0 %
Waitrose	Frozen Mini Macaroni Cheese	1.0 %

Ready Meals - by sugar content (continued)

Brand	Label	% Sugar
Waitrose	Love Life Beef & Red Wine Casserole	1.0 %
Waitrose	Spicy Fusilli with Sausage	1.0 %
Young's	Chip Shop Large Cod Fillet & Chips	1.0 %
ASDA	Chicken & Gravy Large Shortcrust Pastry Pie	1.1 %
ASDA	Chicken Biryani for 2	1.1 %
ASDA	Classic Liver & Bacon with Colcannon Mash	1.1 %
ASDA	Classic Shepherds Pie	1.1 %
ASDA	Classic Shepherd's Pie	1.1 %
ASDA	Extra Special King Prawn Curry with Coconut & Mustard Rice	1.1 %
ASDA	Good & Balanced Moroccan Chicken with Bulgur Wheat	1.1 %
ASDA	Indian Chicken Balti with Pilau Rice	1.1 %
ASDA	Indian Chicken Bhuna with Pilau Rice	1.1 %
ASDA	Italian Chicken & Bacon Pasta Bake	1.1 %
ASDA	Italian Chicken & Bacon Pasta Bake	1.1 %
ASDA	Italian Macaroni Cheese	1.1 %
Birds Eye	Puff Pastry British Steak Pies	1.1 %
Birds Eye	Puff Pastry Chicken & Ham Pies	1.1 %
Bisto	Chicken Hotpot	1.1 %
Cook	Risotto with Porcini Mushrooms, Lemon and Sage Butter	1.1 %
Ginsters	Chicken & Bacon Pasty	1.1 %
Higgidy	Little Smoked Bacon and Cheddar Quiche	1.1 %
Higgidy	Little Spinach & Roasted Red Pepper Quiche	1.1 %
Kingston Town	Curry Mutton with Rice & Gungo Peas	1.1 %

Ready Meals - by sugar content (continued)

Brand	Label	% Sugar
Kirsty's	Beef Lasagne with Rich Bolognese Sauce	1.1 %
Linda McCartney	Cannelloni	1.1 %
Morrisons	Chicken & Bacon Carbonara	1.1 %
Morrisons	Chicken, Ham & Leek Puff Pastry Pie	1.1 %
Morrisons	Dumpling Topped Minced Steak Puff Pastry Pie	1.1 %
Morrisons	M Kitchen Italian Macaroni Cheese	1.1 %
Morrisons	M Kitchen Italian Spaghetti Carbonara	1.1 %
Morrisons	M Kitchen Tastes of Home Cumberland Pie	1.1 %
Morrisons	M Kitchen Tastes of Home Minced Beef Hotpot	1.1 %
Mumtaz	Daal Karahi & Pilau Rice	1.1 %
Our Little Secret	Exotic Seafood Paella	1.1 %
Peter's	Premier Steak & Kidney Pie	1.1 %
Pukka-Pies	Family All Steak Pie	1.1 %
Pukka-Pies	Peppered Steak Pie	1.1 %
Pukka-Pies	Steak & Cheese Pie	1.1 %
Sainsbury's	Classic Shepherd's Pie	1.1 %
Sainsbury's	Pub Specials Chicken in Red Wine & Thyme Sauce	1.1 %
Tesco	Al Fresco Chicken & Roasted Mushrooms	1.1 %
Tesco	Chicken & Mushroom Pie	1.1 %
Tesco	Everyday Value Chicken Curry	1.1 %
Tesco	Everyday Value Macaroni Cheese	1.1 %
Tesco	Family Favourites Cottage Pie	1.1 %
Tesco	Family Favourites Creamy Chicken & Bacon Casserole	1.1 %

Ready Meals - by sugar content (continued)

Brand	Label	% Sugar
Tesco	Finest Chicken & Beech Smoked Bacon Pasta Bake	1.1 %
Tesco	Finest Chicken & Smoked Bacon Pasta Bake	1.1 %
Tesco	Finest Slow Cooked West Country Steak Pie	1.1 %
Tesco	Finest West Country Steak Top Crust Pie	1.1 %
Tesco	Healthy Living Chicken & Bacon Pasta	1.1 %
Tesco	Healthy Living Spaghetti Bolognese	1.1 %
Tesco	Slow Cooked Steak & Kidney Shortcrust Pastry Pie	1.1 %
Tesco	Slow Cooked Steak Shortcrust Pastry Pie	1.1 %
Tesco	Thai Chicken Green Curry with Jasmine Rice	1.1 %
The City Kitchen	Skinny Thai Coconut Chicken	1.1 %
Waitrose	Chicken Forestiere	1.1 %
Waitrose	Cumberland Pie	1.1 %
Waitrose	Macaroni Cheese	1.1 %
Waitrose	Mushroom and Spinach Linguine	1.1 %
Weight Watchers	Chicken Korma with Basmati Rice	1.1 %
Weight Watchers	Red Thai Curry with Jasmine Rice	1.1 %
Tesco	British Classics Chicken Roast Dinner	1.1 %
Tesco	British Classics Sausages & Mash	1.1 %
Tesco	Special Fried Rice	1.1 %
Amy's Kitchen	Bean & Rice Burrito	1.2 %
ASDA	Chicken Singapore Noodles	1.2 %
ASDA	Classic Beef in Peppercorn Sauce	1.2 %
ASDA	Classic Favourites Chicken En Croute	1.2 %

Ready Meals - by sugar content (continued)

Brand	Label	% Sugar
ASDA	Classic Roast Chicken with Peppercorn Sauce	1.2 %
ASDA	Extra Special Beer Battered Cod with Chunky Chips & Pea Puree	1.2 %
ASDA	Extra Special Shepherd's Pie	1.2 %
ASDA	Good & Counted Chinese Chicken Curry & Rice	1.2 %
ASDA	Mini Classics Lamb Hotpot	1.2 %
Aunt Bessie's	Vegetarian Toad in the Hole	1.2 %
Bisto	Minced Beef Hotpot	1.2 %
Cook	Rosemary Chicken with Portobello Mushroom & Pearl Barley Risotto	1.2 %
Fray Bentos	Gentle Minced Beef & Onion Pie	1.2 %
John West	Steam Pot Tuna with Basil and Sun-Dried Tomato Couscous	1.2 %
John West	Steam Pot Tuna with Lemon & Thyme and Tomato & Black Olive Couscous	1.2 %
Morrisons	M Kitchen Tastes of Home Chicken with Leeks, Bacon & Roast Potatoes	1.2 %
Morrisons	Minced Beef & Onion Puff Pastry Pie	1.2 %
Morrisons	Signature Maris Piper Dauphinoise Potatoes	1.2 %
Morrisons	Steak Shortcrust Pie	1.2 %
Peter's	Premier Roast Chicken Pie	1.2 %
Pukka-Pies	Family Chicken & Gravy Pies	1.2 %
Sainsbury's	Chicken Jalfrezi	1.2 %
Tasty Favourites	Chinese Chicken Curry & Rice	1.2 %
Tesco	Chicken & Mushroom Puff Pastry Pie	1.2 %
Tesco	Everyday Value Creamy Mushroom Chicken And Rice	1.2 %
Tesco	Everyday Value Frozen Cottage Pie	1.2 %

Ready Meals – by sugar content (continued)

Brand	Label	% Sugar
Tesco	Everyday Value Minced Beef & Onion Pie	1.2 %
Tesco	Everyday Value Shepherds Pie	1.2 %
Tesco	Family Favourites Carbonara Pasta	1.2 %
Tesco	Modern Italian Chicken Breasts with Creamy Mushroom Sauce	1.2 %
Tesco	Slow Cooked Steak & Ale Puff Pastry Pie	1.2 %
Tesco	Slow Cooked Steak Puff Pastry Pie	1.2 %
Tesco	British Classics Chicken in Mushroom Sauce with Rice	1.2 %
Toscana	Penne Carbonara	1.2 %
Uncle Ben's	Bacon & Mushroom Risotto	1.2 %
Waitrose	Bacon & Pea Risotto	1.2 %
Waitrose	Chicken with Cheese and Bacon	1.2 %
Waitrose	Frozen Chicken & King Prawn Paella	1.2 %
Waitrose	Frozen Green Thai Chicken Noodles	1.2 %
Waitrose	Frozen Mini Sausage & Mash	1.2 %
Waitrose	Love Life Cod in Parsley Sauce	1.2 %
Waitrose	Love Life Creamy Chicken & Vegetable Hotpot	1.2 %
Waitrose	Love Life Ham Hock in Mustard Sauce	1.2 %
Waitrose	Love Life Red Thai Chicken Curry	1.2 %
Waitrose	Menu Chicken Forestiere	1.2 %
Waitrose	Menu Paella	1.2 %
Waitrose	Shepherd's Pie	1.2 %
Weight Watchers From Heinz	Beef Lasagne	1.2 %
ASDA	Bistro Ultimate Steak & Ale Pie	1.3 %

Ready Meals - by sugar content (continued)

Brand	Label	% Sugar
ASDA	Chicken Filled Giant Yorkshire Pudding	1.3 %
ASDA	Chicken in Blackbean Sauce	1.3 %
ASDA	Classic Chicken Breasts in Peppercorn Sauce for 2	1.3 %
ASDA	Classic Favourites Chicken Mini Roasts	1.3 %
ASDA	Classic Haddock Mornay	1.3 %
ASDA	Classic Minced Beef & Dumplings for 2	1.3 %
ASDA	Classic Minced Beef Hot Pot	1.3 %
ASDA	Classic Minced Beef Hotpot for 4	1.3 %
ASDA	Fresh Tastes Kitchen Chicken & Mushroom Risotto	1.3 %
ASDA	Minced Beef & Dumplings for 4	1.3 %
ASDA	Minced Beef Hotpot	1.3 %
ASDA	Singapore Chicken Noodles	1.3 %
ASDA	Smartprice Minced Beef & Dumplings	1.3 %
ASDA	Vegetarian Mushroom Risotto	1.3 %
Charlie Bingham's	Chicken & Mushroom Risotto	1.3 %
Charlie Bingham's	Spaghetti Bolognese	1.3 %
Cook	Lemon Chicken Risotto Family Meal	1.3 %
Cook	Salmon and Asparagus Gratin	1.3 %
Cook	Salmon Wellington	1.3 %
Dolmio	Carbonara Pasta Vista	1.3 %
Dolmio	Creamy Mushroom Pasta Vista	1.3 %
Ginsters	Chicken & Mushroom Pie	1.3 %
Look What We Found!	Tees Valley Beef in Black Velvet Ale	1.3 %

Ready Meals - by sugar content (continued)

Brand	Label	% Sugar
Low Low	Beef Hotpot	1.3 %
Morrisons	Cheese & Onion Small Quiche	1.3 %
Morrisons	Homestyle Lamb Dinner	1.3 %
Morrisons	Just For Kids Bangers & Mash	1.3 %
Morrisons	NuMe Beef in Ale with Mash	1.3 %
Morrisons	NuMe Cumberland Pie	1.3 %
Morrisons	Savers Irish Stew	1.3 %
Mr. Brains	Pork Faggots	1.3 %
Pukka-Pies	Family Steak & Onion Pie	1.3 %
Pukka-Pies	Large Beef and Onion Pie	1.3 %
Sainsbury's	Chicken Korma	1.3 %
Sainsbury's	Pub Specials Chicken & Bacon Risotto	1.3 %
Sainsbury's	Pub Specials Steak & Ale Pies	1.3 %
Tesco	Classic Cumberland Pie	1.3 %
Tesco	Creamy Chicken & Broccoli Large Puff Pastry Pie	1.3 %
Tesco	Creamy Chicken & White Wine Shortcrust Pie	1.3 %
Tesco	Finest Vintage Cheddar Macaroni Cheese	1.3 %
Tesco	Healthy Living Salmon & Broccoli Pie	1.3 %
Tesco	Indian Butter Chicken and Pilau Rice	1.3 %
Tesco	Marinated Chicken with Buttered Courgette Rice	1.3 %
Tesco	Steak & Kidney Pie	1.3 %
Waitrose	Chicken Hotpot	1.3 %
Waitrose	Chicken, White Wine & Tarragon Top Crust Pie	1.3 %
Waitrose	Indian Spinach and Carrot Pilau Rice	1.3 %
Waitrose	Menu Beef Gratin	1.3 %
Waitrose	Tagliatelle with Ham	1.3 %

Ready Meals - by sugar content (continued)

Brand	Label	% Sugar
Weight Watchers	Chicken, Tomato & Spinach Lasagne	1.3 %
Weight Watchers	Classic Cottage Pie	1.3 %
Young's	Gastro Pink Salmon, Alaska Pollock & Cherry Tomato Bake	1.3 %
Tesco	British Classics Chicken Casserole & Dumplings	1.3 %
Tesco	British Classics Cottage Pie	1.3 %
Tesco	British Classics Large Fish Pie	1.3 %
Tesco	British Classics Turkey Roast Dinner	1.3 %
Tesco	Oriental Chicken Chow Mein	1.4 %
ASDA	Cheese & Onion Pie	1.4 %
ASDA	Chinese Chicken Chop Suey with Egg Fried Rice	1.4 %
ASDA	Classic Chicken Hotpot	1.4 %
ASDA	Classic Chicken, Leek & Bacon Bake	1.4 %
ASDA	Classic Minced Beef Hot Pot for 2	1.4 %
ASDA	Good & Counted Chicken Tikka Masala with Pilau Rice	1.4 %
ASDA	Good & Counted Cottage Pie	1.4 %
ASDA	Mini Classics Chicken Hotpot	1.4 %
ASDA	Roast Beef Dinner	1.4 %
ASDA	Sausage & Onion Shortcrust Pie	1.4 %
ASDA	Vegetarian Chilli Burrito	1.4 %
Birds Eye	Four Cheese Penne Pasta	1.4 %
Bisto	Roast Lamb Dinner	1.4 %
Charlie Bingham's	Chilli con Carne & Mexican Rice	1.4 %

Ready Meals - by sugar content (continued)

Brand	Label	% Sugar
Charlie Bingham's	Cottage Pie	1.4 %
John West	Steam Pot Tuna with Mixed Peppercorn and Tomato & Black Olive Couscous	1.4 %
Kirsty's	Sausage And Sweet Potato Mash	1.4 %
Linda McCartney	Farmhouse Pies	1.4 %
Look What We Found!	Tees Valley Beef Casserole	1.4 %
Morrisons	M Kitchen Fresh Ideas Honey & Mustard Chicken	1.4 %
Morrisons	M Kitchen Fresh Ideas Tandoori Chicken	1.4 %
Morrisons	M Kitchen Italian Beef Lasagne	1.4 %
Morrisons	M Kitchen Italian Bolognese Pasta Bake	1.4 %
Morrisons	M Kitchen Oriental Special Chicken Fried Rice	1.4 %
Morrisons	M Kitchen Tastes of Home Chicken Dinner with Stuffing	1.4 %
Morrisons	M Kitchen Tastes of Home Corned Beef Hatch	1.4 %
Morrisons	Minced Steak & Onion Shortcrust Pie	1.4 %
Morrisons	Signature Maple-Cured Bacon & Gruyere Tart	1.4 %
Morrisons	Signature Wild Mushroom & West Country Cheddar Tart	1.4 %
Pieminister	Matador Pie	1.4 %
Quorn	Meat Free Chicken Style & Mushroom Pie	1.4 %
Quorn	Meat Free Cottage Pie	1.4 %
Sainsbury's	Basics Beef Curry with Rice	1.4 %
Sainsbury's	Classic Chicken Dinner	1.4 %
Tesco	Beef Curry	1.4 %

Ready Meals - by sugar content (continued)

Brand	Label	% Sugar
Tesco	Big Night In Indian Tarka Dahl	1.4 %
Tesco	Chicken & Ham Puff Pastry Lattice	1.4 %
Tesco	Classic Chicken Dinner	1.4 %
Tesco	Classic Italian Chicken & Bacon Pasta Bake	1.4 %
Tesco	Classic Italian Spaghetti Carbonara	1.4 %
Tesco	Everyday Value Chicken & Gravy Pie	1.4 %
Tesco	Everyday Value Chicken Hotpot	1.4 %
Tesco	Everyday Value Minced Beef & Onion Pies	1.4 %
Tesco	Family Favourites Minced Beef with Potatoes	1.4 %
Tesco	Indian Tarka Dahl	1.4 %
Tesco	Minced Beef & Onion Pie	1.4 %
Tesco	Modern Italian Spicy Beef & Jalapeno Melt	1.4 %
Tesco	Oriental Green Thai Chicken Curry with Rice	1.4 %
Tesco	Spinach & Ricotta Puff Pastry Tart	1.4 %
Tesco	Steak Pie	1.4 %
Waitrose	Bubble & Squeak	1.4 %
Waitrose	Crustless Spinach, Feta and Roasted Red Pepper Quiche	1.4 %
Waitrose	Love Life Green Thai Chicken Curry	1.4 %
Waitrose	Love Life Piri Piri Chicken	1.4 %
Waitrose	Menu Cottage Pie	1.4 %
Waitrose	Roast Chicken Large Pie	1.4 %
Weight Watchers	Chicken Tikka with Basmati Rice	1.4 %
Weight Watchers From Heinz	Cottage Pie	1.4 %

Ready Meals - by sugar content (continued)

Brand	Label	% Sugar
Amy's Kitchen	Gluten Free Black Bean & Vegetable Enchilada	1.5 %
ASDA	Chef's Special Singapore Noodles	1.5 %
ASDA	Chicken Curry Pies	1.5 %
ASDA	Classic Chicken, Leek & Bacon Bake for 2	1.5 %
ASDA	Classic Sausages & Mash	1.5 %
ASDA	Good & Counted Fish Pie	1.5 %
ASDA	Italian Beef Bolognese Pasta Bake	1.5 %
ASDA	Italian Ham & Mushroom Tagliatelle	1.5 %
ASDA	Pub Classics Peppercorn Chicken with Sautéed Potatoes	1.5 %
ASDA	Smart Price Minced Beef & Onion Pies	1.5 %
ASDA	Smartprice Chicken Curry & Rice	1.5 %
ASDA	Smartprice Spaghetti Carbonara	1.5 %
ASDA	Vegetarian Spicy Three Bean Enchiladas	1.5 %
Birds Eye	Prawn Curry with Rice	1.5 %
Birds Eye	Shortcrust Meat & Potato Pies	1.5 %
Birds Eye	Shortcrust Steak Pies	1.5 %
Birds Eye	Stir Your Senses South Indian Chicken Curry	1.5 %
Birds Eye	Stir Your Senses Tagliatelle con Porcini	1.5 %
Birds Eye	Stir Your Senses Thai Chicken with Basmati Rice	1.5 %
Birds Eye	Traditional Beef Dinner	1.5 %
Bisto	Roast Beef Dinner	1.5 %
Bisto	Roast Chicken Dinner	1.5 %
Charlie Bingham's	Fish Pie	1.5 %
Cook	Liver, Bacon and Onions	1.5 %

Ready Meals – by sugar content (continued)

Brand	Label	% Sugar
Ginsters	Steak & Kidney Pie	1.5 %
Heinz	Big Chicken Casserole with Chunky Potatoes	1.5 %
Higgidy	Spinach, Feta & Toasted Pine Nut Pie	1.5 %
Holland's	Guinness Steak Pie	1.5 %
Holland's	Meat Pies	1.5 %
John West	Steam Pot Tuna with Coriander & Cumin and Thyme & Coriander Couscous	1.5 %
Morrisons	M Kitchen Italian Bolognese Pasta Melt	1.5 %
Morrisons	M Kitchen Italian Spaghetti Bolognese	1.5 %
Morrisons	M Kitchen Tastes of Home Roast Chicken Dinner	1.5 %
Morrisons	M Kitchen Tastes of Home Shepherd's Pie	1.5 %
Morrisons	Macaroni Cheese	1.5 %
Morrisons	Quiche Lorraine	1.5 %
Morrisons	Savers Macaroni Cheese	1.5 %
Mumtaz	Keema Mattar Karahi & Pilau Rice	1.5 %
Princes	Creamy Cheese Tuna Pasta Bake	1.5 %
Pukka-Pies	Large All Steak Pie	1.5 %
Sainsbury's	Basics Beef In Gravy	1.5 %
Sainsbury's	Basics Macaroni Cheese	1.5 %
Sainsbury's	Classic Chicken Hotpot Dinner	1.5 %
Sainsbury's	Pub Specials Gammon Hock in a Cider Sauce with Mustard Mash	1.5 %
Sharwood's	Chinese Chicken Curry with Rice	1.5 %
Tasty Favourites	Beef Hot Pot	1.5 %
Tesco	Classic Italian Chicken & Bacon Pasta Bake	1.5 %
Tesco	Classic Italian Ham & Mushroom Tagliatelle	1.5 %

Ready Meals – by sugar content (continued)

Brand	Label	% Sugar
Tesco	Classic Italian Spaghetti Bolognese	1.5 %
Tesco	Creamy Chicken & Bacon Large Puff Pastry Pie	1.5 %
Tesco	Finest Chicken Biriyani	1.5 %
Tesco	Finest Traditional Lasagne	1.5 %
Tesco	Healthy Living Chicken & Broccoli Pie	1.5 %
Tesco	British Classics Chicken in Red Wine Sauce with Rosemary Potatoes	1.5 %
Tesco	British Classics Cumberland Pie	1.5 %
Tesco	British Classics Minced Beef Hotpot	1.5 %
The City Kitchen	Malaysian Coconut Beef Curry	1.5 %
Waitrose	Frozen Chicken Biryani	1.5 %
Waitrose	Frozen Mini Liver & Bacon	1.5 %
Waitrose	Vegetable Chilli with Rice	1.5 %
Weight Watchers	Spanish Chicken & Patatas Bravas	1.5 %
Amy's Kitchen	Gluten Free Cheese Enchilada	1.6 %
ASDA	Chicken & Asparagus Large Puff Pastry Pie	1.6 %
ASDA	Chicken Madras with Pilau Rice	1.6 %
ASDA	Extra Special Lamb Hotpot with Wainwright Ale	1.6 %
ASDA	Family Size Deep Filled Slow-Cooked Steak & Gravy Pie	1.6 %
ASDA	Fresh Tastes Kitchen Chicken & Bacon Carbonara	1.6 %
ASDA	Good & Balanced Chicken Tikka & Aubergine Dahl	1.6 %
ASDA	Good & Balanced Seafood Paella	1.6 %
ASDA	Good & Counted Tuna Pasta Bake	1.6 %

Ready Meals - by sugar content (continued)

Brand	Label	% Sugar
ASDA	Italian Chicken & Mushroom Tagliatelle	1.6 %
ASDA	Italian Spaghetti Carbonara	1.6 %
ASDA	Mini Classics Fish Pie	1.6 %
ASDA	Pasta Carbonara for 4	1.6 %
ASDA	Steak & Gravy Large Puff Pastry Pie	1.6 %
ASDA	Steak & Potato Puff Pastry Plait	1.6 %
ASDA	Taste of America Homestyle Beefy Chilli & Rice	1.6 %
ASDA	Taste of America Mighty Fine Blue Cheese Mac & Bacon	1.6 %
Morrisons	Cheese & Broccoli Quiche	1.6 %
Morrisons	Homestyle Chicken Dinner	1.6 %
Morrisons	Just For Kids Chicken Dinner	1.6 %
Morrisons	M Kitchen Chicken Tikka Biryani	1.6 %
Morrisons	M Kitchen Fresh Ideas Piri Piri Chicken	1.6 %
Morrisons	M Kitchen Italian Lasagne	1.6 %
Morrisons	M Kitchen Tastes of Home Roast Beef Dinner	1.6 %
Morrisons	Quiche Lorraine Small	1.6 %
Morrisons	Savers Cheese & Onion Quiche	1.6 %
Morrisons	Tomato & Cheese Crustless Quiche	1.6 %
Pieminister	Chicken of Aragon Pie	1.6 %
Pukka-Pies	Frozen Family Chicken & Veg Pies	1.6 %
Pukka-Pies	Frozen Family Steak Pies	1.6 %
Pukka-Pies	Minced Steak & Onion Pies	1.6 %
Quorn	Meat Free Curry & Rice	1.6 %
Sainsbury's	Chickpea Dahl	1.6 %
Sainsbury's	Classic Gammon & Parsley Sauce	1.6 %

Ready Meals - by sugar content (continued)

Brand	Label	% Sugar
Sainsbury's	Pub Specials Creamy Peppercorn Chicken	1.6 %
Smart-GF Kids	Kooky Korma	1.6 %
Tasty Favourites	Chilli Con Carne	1.6 %
Tesco	Chicken & Gravy Shortcrust Pie	1.6 %
Tesco	Chicken, Bacon & Cheese Bakes	1.6 %
Tesco	Creamy Chicken Bakes	1.6 %
Tesco	Everyday Value Cheese Burger And Chips	1.6 %
Tesco	Finest Chicken in a White Wine Sauce with Leeks	1.6 %
Tesco	Healthy Living Cottage Pie	1.6 %
Tesco	Slow Cooked Minced Steak & Onion Shortcrust Pastry Pie	1.6 %
Tesco	British Classics Braised Beef & Mash	1.6 %
Tesco	British Classics Chicken & Stuffing Bake	1.6 %
Tesco	British Classics Liver, Bacon & Mash	1.6 %
Waitrose	Chicken Tagliatelle	1.6 %
Waitrose	Chicken, Leek & White Wine Large Pie	1.6 %
Waitrose	Filled Jacket Potatoes	1.6 %
Waitrose	Indian Spinach Dal	1.6 %
Waitrose	Love Life Pea & Spinach Open Ravioli	1.6 %
Waitrose	Menu Beef Stroganoff	1.6 %
Waitrose	Menu Ham Hock & Camembert Crepes	1.6 %
Waitrose	Spinach Mornay	1.6 %
ASDA	Chef's Special Kerala Beef & Black Pepper Sauce	1.7 %
ASDA	Chicken Korma with Pilau Rice	1.7 %

Ready Meals - by sugar content (continued)

Brand	Label	% Sugar
ASDA	Chinese Chicken Curry with Egg Fried Rice	1.7 %
ASDA	Extra Special Lamb Moussaka for 2	1.7 %
ASDA	Fresh Tastes Kitchen Chinese Chicken Curry & Rice	1.7 %
ASDA	Indian Scorching Hot Chicken Vindaloo with Pilau Rice	1.7 %
ASDA	Italian Spaghetti Bolognese	1.7 %
ASDA	Italian Three Cheese & Tomato Pasta Bake	1.7 %
ASDA	Italian Three Cheese & Tomato Pasta Bake for 2	1.7 %
ASDA	Mexican Chilli & Rice for 4	1.7 %
ASDA	Pub Classics Boozy Beef Pie	1.7 %
ASDA	Smartprice Cottage Pie	1.7 %
ASDA	Vegetable & Cheese Pies	1.7 %
Charlie Bingham's	Chicken Jalfrezi & Pilau Rice	1.7 %
Cook	Chicken Alexander	1.7 %
Cook	Coq au Vin	1.7 %
Cook	Sea Bass with Asparagus & Linguine in Lobster & Saffron Bisque	1.7 %
Hungry Joe's	Blazin' Beef Chilli & Spicy Rice	1.7 %
Look What We Found!	Chilli Con Carne & Long Grain Rice	1.7 %
Morrisons	Classic Sausage & Chips	1.7 %
Morrisons	M Kitchen Tastes of Home Potato Gratin	1.7 %
Morrisons	M Kitchen Tex Mex Family Chilli Con Carne & Rice	1.7 %
Morrisons	Savers Cheese & Bacon Quiche	1.7 %
Morrisons	Steak & Kidney Shortcrust Pie	1.7 %

Ready Meals – by sugar content (continued)

Brand	Label	% Sugar
Princes	Hot Chicken Curry	1.7 %
Pukka-Pies	Large Chicken Balti Pie	1.7 %
Pukka-Pies	Large Potato, Cheese & Onion Pie	1.7 %
Pukka-Pies	Microwaveable All Steak Pie	1.7 %
Pukka-Pies	Steak & Kidney Pudding	1.7 %
Quorn	Meat Free Low Fat Sausages	1.7 %
Sainsbury's	Chicken Balti	1.7 %
Sharwood's	Lamb Biryani	1.7 %
Tesco	Al Fresco Pulled Pork in Cannellini Bean Sauce	1.7 %
Tesco	Big Night In Thai Green Chicken Curry & Jasmine Rice	1.7 %
Tesco	Chicken & Gravy Shortcrust Pastry Pie	1.7 %
Tesco	Chicken, Ham Hock, & Leek Puff Pastry Pies	1.7 %
Tesco	Classic Beef Dinner	1.7 %
Tesco	Creamy Chicken & White Wine Large Shortcrust Pie	1.7 %
Tesco	Everyday Value Spaghetti Bolognese	1.7 %
Tesco	Finest Lemon & Black Pepper Chicken Pasta	1.7 %
Tesco	Finest Spaghetti Bolognese	1.7 %
Tesco	Healthy Living Chicken & Prawn Paella	1.7 %
Tesco	Modern Italian Chilli Beef Lasagne	1.7 %
Tesco	Slow Cooked Steak & Onion Puff Pastry Lattice	1.7 %
Tesco	Slow Cooked Steak & Onion Puff Pastry Pie	1.7 %
Tesco	Slow Cooked Steak Shortcrust Pastry Pie	1.7 %
Tesco	Big Night In Chinese Chicken Chow Mein	1.7 %
Tesco	Takeaway No 25 Vegetable Chop Suey	1.7 %

Ready Meals - by sugar content (continued)

Brand	Label	% Sugar
The City Kitchen	Malaysian Chicken Curry Noodles	1.7 %
Waitrose	Menu Quiche Lorraine	1.7 %
Waitrose	Menu Smoked Fish Gratin	1.7 %
Waitrose	Steak Large Pie	1.7 %
Weight Watchers	Cheese & Onion Crustless Quiche	1.7 %
Weight Watchers	Macaroni Cheese	1.7 %
Weight Watchers From Heinz	Beef Hotpot	1.7 %
Weight Watchers From Heinz	Chicken In White Wine Sauce	1.7 %
ASDA	Chinese Chicken Chow Mein	1.8 %
ASDA	Chinese Chicken in Blackbean Sauce	1.8 %
ASDA	Classic Liver & Bacon with Mashed	1.8 %
ASDA	Express Meals Chicken Paella	1.8 %
ASDA	Fresh Tastes Kitchen Chicken & Mushroom Stroganoff	1.8 %
ASDA	Italian Beef Bolognese Pasta Bake for 2	1.8 %
ASDA	Italian King Prawn Linguine	1.8 %
ASDA	Kids Bangers & Mash	1.8 %
ASDA	Kids Lamb Hotpot	1.8 %
ASDA	Pub Classics Gammon & Mash	1.8 %
ASDA	Salmon & Broccoli Puff Pastry Lattice	1.8 %
ASDA	Smartprice Macaroni Cheese	1.8 %

Ready Meals - by sugar content (continued)

Brand	Label	% Sugar
ASDA	Taste of America Finger Lickin' Southern Fried Chicken & Spicy Wedges	1.8 %
ASDA	Taste of America Mucho Gusto Meatballs & Herby Rice	1.8 %
Aunt Bessie's	Deep Filled Chicken Pie	1.8 %
Aunt Bessie's	Large Toad in the Hole	1.8 %
Birds Eye	Creamy Cheese Penne Pasta	1.8 %
Birds Eye	Shortcrust Chicken Pies	1.8 %
Birds Eye	Steamfresh Creamy Cheese Penne Pasta	1.8 %
Birds Eye	Stir Your Senses Rigatoni alla Carbonara	1.8 %
Cook	Slow-cooked Rump Beef with Brandy	1.8 %
Cook	Thai Style Chicken Patties	1.8 %
Ginsters	Original Cornish Pasty	1.8 %
Higgidy	Cauliflower Cheese Pie with Chestnut Crumble	1.8 %
John West	Light Lunch Italian Style Tuna Salad	1.8 %
Little Dish	Fisherman's Pie with Salmon and Pollock	1.8 %
Morrisons	Cheese & Onion Crustless Quiche	1.8 %
Morrisons	Just for Kids Cottage Pie	1.8 %
Morrisons	M Kitchen Fresh Ideas Mexican Chicken	1.8 %
Morrisons	M Kitchen Indian Chicken Pasanda & Pilau Rice	1.8 %
Morrisons	M Kitchen Italian Chicken & Bacon Pasta Bake	1.8 %
Morrisons	M Kitchen Tastes of Home Minced Lamb Casserole	1.8 %
Morrisons	M Kitchen Vegetarian Vegetable Pasta Bake	1.8 %
Morrisons	Signature Cauliflower Cheese with Davidstow Cheddar	1.8 %
Pieminister	The Deerstalker Pie	1.8 %

Ready Meals – by sugar content (continued)

Brand	Label	% Sugar
Pooles	Potato & Meat Pies	1.8 %
Pukka-Pies	Chicken & Vegetable Pies	1.8 %
Quorn	Meat Free Italian Pasta Bake	1.8 %
Sainsbury's	Be Good Chicken Curry with Rice	1.8 %
Sainsbury's	Be Good Lemon Chicken Risotto	1.8 %
Sainsbury's	Chicken & Mushroom Pies	1.8 %
Sainsbury's	Steak & Kidney Pies	1.8 %
Tesco	Chicken & Bacon Pies	1.8 %
Tesco	Classic Italian Large Beef Lasagne	1.8 %
Tesco	Everyday Value Minced Beef Hotpot	1.8 %
Tesco	Finest Lasagne Al Forno	1.8 %
Tesco	Finest Smoked Haddock Fishcakes	1.8 %
Tesco	Healthy Living Baked Potatoes with Cheese	1.8 %
Tesco	Healthy Living Chilli & Rice	1.8 %
Tesco	Modern Italian Creamy Prawn Linguine	1.8 %
Tesco	Slow Cooked Minced Steak & Onion Large Shortcrust Pastry Pie	1.8 %
Tesco	Steak & Ale Puff Pastry Pies	1.8 %
Tesco	Toad In The Hole	1.8 %
The City Kitchen	Vegetables with Coconut & Lentil Pilaf	1.8 %
Waitrose	Chicken & Chorizo Paella	1.8 %
Waitrose	Chicken Pie	1.8 %
Waitrose	Chicken Provençal	1.8 %
Waitrose	Cod Fillet in Parsley Sauce	1.8 %
Waitrose	Delisante Artisan Salmon & Watercress Quiche	1.8 %
Waitrose	Frozen Roast Chicken Pies	1.8 %

Ready Meals - by sugar content (continued)

Brand	Label	% Sugar
Waitrose	Garlic Mushroom Gratin	1.8 %
Waitrose	Indian Tarka Dahl	1.8 %
Waitrose	Love Life Roasted Mushroom Risotto	1.8 %
Waitrose	Orkney Crab Gratin	1.8 %
Waitrose	Spinach Cannelloni	1.8 %
Weight Watchers	Chicken Jambalaya	1.8 %
Amy's Kitchen	Gluten Free Bean & Rice Burrito	1.9 %
Amy's Kitchen	Gluten Free Cheddar, Rice & Bean Burrito	1.9 %
Amy's Kitchen	Vegetable Lasagne	1.9 %
ASDA	Cheese & Onion Bakes	1.9 %
ASDA	Chicken & Mushroom Pies	1.9 %
ASDA	Chicken Hotpot	1.9 %
ASDA	Chicken in Red Wine with Creamy Garlic Potatoes	1.9 %
ASDA	Classic Beef Goulash & Dumplings	1.9 %
ASDA	Deep Filled Roast Chicken Pie	1.9 %
ASDA	Extra Special Four Cheese Macaroni	1.9 %
ASDA	Extra Special Lamb Moussaka for 1	1.9 %
ASDA	Fish Pie	1.9 %
ASDA	Good & Counted Tomato & Mascarpone Pasta Bake	1.9 %
ASDA	Italian Pepperoni Pasta Bake	1.9 %
ASDA	Mini Classics Beef Stew & Dumpling	1.9 %
Birds Eye	Stir Your Senses Pappardelle alla Bolognese	1.9 %
Bisto	Beef Lasagne	1.9 %
Bisto	Roast Turkey Dinner	1.9 %

Ready Meals - by sugar content (continued)

Brand	Label	% Sugar
Cauldron	South American Empanadas	1.9 %
Charlie Bingham's	Shepherd's Pie	1.9 %
Charlie Bingham's	Spaghetti Carbonara	1.9 %
Cook	Beef Stroganoff	1.9 %
Cook	Chicken & Pancetta Pie	1.9 %
Fray Bentos	Hunger Burster Beef Stew & Dumplings	1.9 %
Genius	Gluten Free Chicken & Gravy Pies	1.9 %
Heinz	Big Chilli Con Carne with Chunky Wedges	1.9 %
Heinz	Big Pasta Bolognese with Chunky Pasta	1.9 %
Little Dish	Chicken and Butternut Squash Pie	1.9 %
Little Dish	Chunky Chicken Pot Roast	1.9 %
Little Dish	Mild Beef Chilli & Rice	1.9 %
Morrisons	Bacon & Leek Small Quiche	1.9 %
Morrisons	Classic Steak let & Chips	1.9 %
Morrisons	M Kitchen Indian Chicken Madras & Pilau Rice	1.9 %
Morrisons	M Kitchen Tex Mex Chilli Beef Burrito	1.9 %
Morrisons	NuMe Chicken Tikka Masala & Pilau Rice	1.9 %
Pieminister	Fungi Chicken Pie	1.9 %
Sainsbury's	Basics Chicken & Vegetable Pies	1.9 %
Sainsbury's	Basics Chicken Curry with Rice	1.9 %
Sainsbury's	Basics Minced Beef Hotpot	1.9 %
Tasty Favourites	Chicken Korma	1.9 %
Tesco	Al Fresco Pea & Pancetta Risotto	1.9 %
Tesco	Big Night In Thai Red Chicken Curry & Rice	1.9 %

Ready Meals - by sugar content (continued)

Brand	Label	% Sugar
Tesco	Cheese & Bacon Crustless Quiche	1.9 %
Tesco	Chicken & Vegetable Pies	1.9 %
Tesco	Finest Chicken Dhansak with Pilau Rice	1.9 %
Tesco	Finest Potato Topped Chicken Pie	1.9 %
Tesco	Finest Roast Chicken & Italian Pancetta Bake	1.9 %
Tesco	Oriental Red Thai Chicken Curry with Rice	1.9 %
Tesco	Oriental Chicken & Mushroom With Egg Fried Rice	1.9 %
The City Kitchen	Skinny Bombay Spiced Chicken	1.9 %
The City Kitchen	Takeaway No 65 Singapore Noodles	1.9 %
Waitrose	Cajun Chicken Tagliatelle	1.9 %
Waitrose	Menu Shepherd's Pie	1.9 %
Waitrose	Piri Piri Chicken	1.9 %
Waitrose	Quiche Lorraine	1.9 %
Waitrose	Rigatoni and Aubergine	1.9 %
Waitrose	Steak & Stout Pie	1.9 %
Weight Watchers From Heinz	Ocean Pie	1.9 %
Young's	Admiral's Pie	1.9 %
ASDA	Chicken Curried Rice	2.0 %
ASDA	Chicken Jalfrezi with Pilau Rice	2.0 %
ASDA	Chicken Korma	2.0 %
ASDA	Extra Special Chicken, Chorizo & King Prawn Paella	2.0 %
ASDA	Extra Special Spicy Chilli Steak & Rice	2.0 %

Ready Meals - by sugar content (continued)

Brand	Label	% Sugar
ASDA	Fresh Tastes Kitchen Chicken Chow Mein	2.0 %
ASDA	Fresh Tastes Kitchen Ham Hock with Potatoes	2.0 %
ASDA	Good & Counted Cottage Pie	2.0 %
ASDA	Italian Beef Cannelloni	2.0 %
ASDA	Italian Chicken Tagliatelle	2.0 %
ASDA	Italian Meatball Pasta Bake for 2	2.0 %
ASDA	Kids Spaghetti Bolognese	2.0 %
Aunt Bessie's	Deep Filled Steak Pie	2.0 %
Aunt Bessie's	Toad in the Hole	2.0 %
Birds Eye	Macaroni with Cheese & Ham	2.0 %
Birds Eye	Shortcrust Creamy Chicken Pies	2.0 %
Charlie Bingham's	Macaroni Cheese	2.0 %
Charlie Bingham's	Spanish Chicken & Roasted Potatoes	2.0 %
Charlie Bingham's	Thai Green Chicken Curry	2.0 %
Cook	Chicken, Ham and Leek Pie	2.0 %
Cook	Kids Cottage Pie	2.0 %
Cook	Lamb Casserole with New Potatoes	2.0 %
Cook	Spaghetti Bolognese	2.0 %
Cook	Steak and Red Wine Pie	2.0 %
Easy Bean	African Palava	2.0 %
John West	Steam Pot Tuna with Soy & Ginger and Mushroom Couscous	2.0 %
Linda McCartney	Mushroom and Ale Pie	2.0 %

Ready Meals - by sugar content (continued)

Brand	Label	% Sugar
Look What We Found!	Staffordshire Chicken Korma	2.0 %
Morrisons	Homestyle Liver & Onions	2.0 %
Morrisons	M Kitchen Oriental Green Thai Chicken Curry with Jasmine Rice	2.0 %
Morrisons	M Kitchen Tastes of Home Slow-Cooked Lamb Shank with Mint Gravy	2.0 %
Morrisons	Signature Brie & Pancetta Tart	2.0 %
Morrisons	Signature British Lamb Moussaka	2.0 %
Morrisons	Spinach & Ricotta Quiche	2.0 %
Pieminister	Cheeky Chick Pie Pot	2.0 %
Princes	Mild Chicken Curry	2.0 %
Pukka-Pies	Beef and Onion Pukka Pasty	2.0 %
Quorn	Meat Free Chef's Selection Steak & Gravy Pudding	2.0 %
Quorn	Meat Free Steak Style Slice	2.0 %
Quorn	Meat Free Stew & Dumplings	2.0 %
Sainsbury's	Classic Beef Dinner	2.0 %
Sharwood's	Chicken Korma with Rice	2.0 %
Tesco	Big Night In Indian Saag Aloo	2.0 %
Tesco	Chicken Tikka Masala	2.0 %
Tesco	Classic Italian Beef Lasagne	2.0 %
Tesco	Classic Lamb Hotpot	2.0 %
Tesco	Everyday Value Chicken Vegetable Pies	2.0 %
Tesco	Everyday Value Toad In The Hole	2.0 %
Tesco	Finest Chicken Chasseur	2.0 %
Tesco	Finest Lamb Rogan Josh with Pilau Rice	2.0 %

Ready Meals - by sugar content (continued)

Brand	Label	% Sugar
Tesco	Indian Saag Aloo	2.0 %
Tesco	Lamb Rogan Josh	2.0 %
Tesco	Small Quiche Lorraine	2.0 %
Tesco	Al Fresco Beef Stifado with Chunky Potatoes	2.0 %
Waitrose	Broccoli & Gruyère Quiche	2.0 %
Waitrose	Chicken, Ham Hock & Leek Pie	2.0 %
Waitrose	Frozen Mini Chicken Dinner	2.0 %
Waitrose	Frozen Seafood Risotto	2.0 %
Waitrose	Frozen Steak & Ale Pies	2.0 %
Waitrose	Ham Hock in Cider & Mustard Sauce	2.0 %
Waitrose	Love Life Harissa Chicken	2.0 %
Waitrose	Love Life Smoky Chorizo Chicken	2.0 %
Waitrose	Menu Mushroom Open Ravioli	2.0 %
Waitrose	Steak & Kidney Puddings	2.0 %
Weight Watchers From Heinz	Spaghetti Bolognese	2.0 %
Weight Watchers From Heinz	Thai Green Chicken Curry	2.0 %
Young's	Fisherman's Pie	2.0 %
Young's	Ocean Pie	2.0 %
Amy's Kitchen	Gluten Free Broccoli & Cheddar Bake	2.1 %
ASDA	Chicken Casserole for 4	2.1 %
ASDA	Chicken Chow Mein	2.1 %
ASDA	Classic All Day Breakfast	2.1 %
ASDA	Classic Chicken Pie & Mash	2.1 %

Ready Meals – by sugar content (continued)

Brand	Label	% Sugar
ASDA	Extra Special Spaghetti Bolognese	2.1 %
ASDA	Extra Special West Country Beef Bourguignon	2.1 %
ASDA	Family Favourites Beef Lasagne	2.1 %
ASDA	Fresh Tastes Kitchen Chicken & King Prawn Paella	2.1 %
ASDA	Fresh Tastes Kitchen Pad Thai Chicken Noodles	2.1 %
ASDA	Fresh Tastes Kitchen Spicy Chicken & Chorizo Pasta	2.1 %
ASDA	Good & Counted Beef Chilli & Rice	2.1 %
ASDA	Good & Counted Chicken Hotpot	2.1 %
ASDA	Good & Counted Chicken Nacho Bake with Potato Wedges	2.1 %
ASDA	Italian Chicken Lasagne	2.1 %
ASDA	Kids Chicken & Butternut Squash Risotto	2.1 %
ASDA	Kids Pasta Bolognese	2.1 %
ASDA	Kids Spaghetti & Meatballs	2.1 %
ASDA	Loaded Spicy Pepperoni Pasta Bake Meal for 2	2.1 %
ASDA	Mini Classics Chilli & Rice	2.1 %
ASDA	Smartprice Lasagne for 4	2.1 %
ASDA	Taste of America Kickin' Chicken Enchiladas	2.1 %
Bisto	Toad In The Hole	2.1 %
Cook	Kids Chicken and Mash Pie	2.1 %
Cook	Nasi Goreng For 2	2.1 %
Cook	Pot Roast Chicken	2.1 %
Cook	Steak, Mushroom & Merlot Pie	2.1 %
Holland's	Pub Classics Chicken & Ham Pie	2.1 %

Ready Meals - by sugar content (continued)

Brand	Label	% Sugar
Levi Roots	Jamaican Coconut Chicken Curry with Rice & Peas	2.1 %
Little Dish	Mediterranean Cod and Tomato Casserole	2.1 %
Low Low	Chicken in White Wine Sauce with Pasta	2.1 %
Morrisons	Homestyle Beef Dinner	2.1 %
Morrisons	Just For Kids Chicken Casserole	2.1 %
Morrisons	M Kitchen Oriental Chicken Chow Mein	2.1 %
Morrisons	NuMe Cheese & Onion Quiche	2.1 %
Morrisons	Quiche Lorraine Crustless	2.1 %
Morrisons	Signature Shepherd's Pie with Leeks	2.1 %
Morrisons	Tomato, Bacon & Mushroom Quiche	2.1 %
Pieminister	Wild Shroom Pie	2.1 %
Pooles	Cheese & Onion Pies	2.1 %
Sainsbury's	Basics Chilli con Carne with Rice	2.1 %
Sainsbury's	Be Good Beef Lasagne	2.1 %
Sharwood's	Chicken Chow Mein	2.1 %
Tasty Favourites	Bolognese Pasta	2.1 %
Tesco	Bacon & Leek Quiche	2.1 %
Tesco	Big Night In Indian Chicken Biryani	2.1 %
Tesco	Chinese Chicken Curried Rice	2.1 %
Tesco	Classic Minced Beef Filled Yorkshire	2.1 %
Tesco	Everyday Value Macaroni Cheese	2.1 %
Tesco	Finest Beef Chianti with Rosemary Potatoes	2.1 %
Tesco	Finest Beef In Chianti with Potatoes	2.1 %
Tesco	Finest Chicken Tikka Masala & Jalfrezi Meal For 2	2.1 %

Ready Meals - by sugar content (continued)

Brand	Label	% Sugar
Tesco	Finest Large Lasagne Al Forno	2.1 %
Tesco	Finest Prawn Tikka Masala with Pilau Rice	2.1 %
Tesco	Healthy Living Chicken with Baby Potatoes & Vegetables	2.1 %
Tesco	Indian Chicken Korma and Pilau Rice	2.1 %
Tesco	Indian Chicken Tikka Masala With Pilau Rice	2.1 %
Tesco	Oriental Chicken & Blackbean With Egg Fried Rice	2.1 %
Waitrose	Frozen Mini Spaghetti Bolognese	2.1 %
Waitrose	Frozen Steak & Mushroom Pies	2.1 %
Waitrose	Lamb Hotpot	2.1 %
Waitrose	Quiche Lorraine Small	2.1 %
Waitrose	Steak, Mushroom & Red Wine Pie	2.1 %
Amy's Kitchen	Gluten Free Mexican Tortilla Bake	2.2 %
Annabel Karmel	Scrummy Chicken & Rice	2.2 %
ASDA	Chicken & Vegetable Pies	2.2 %
ASDA	Chicken Chow Mein	2.2 %
ASDA	Chicken Curry Bakes	2.2 %
ASDA	Classic Beef & Ale Stew with Dumplings	2.2 %
ASDA	Fresh Tastes Kitchen Roast Chicken Dinner	2.2 %
ASDA	Good & Balanced Chicken & Roasted Butternut Squash Pasta	2.2 %
ASDA	Good & Counted Chicken Chow Mein	2.2 %
ASDA	Indian Chicken Tikka Masala with Pilau Rice	2.2 %
ASDA	Italian Chilli Beef Pasta Bake for 2	2.2 %
ASDA	Kids Cottage Pie	2.2 %

Ready Meals - by sugar content (continued)

Brand	Label	% Sugar
ASDA	Kids Fish Pie	2.2 %
Birds Eye	Chicken Curry with Rice	2.2 %
Birds Eye	Chicken Jalfrezi with Rice	2.2 %
Birds Eye	Chicken Tikka Masala with Rice	2.2 %
Charlie Bingham's	Chicken Korma & Pilau Rice	2.2 %
Charlie Bingham's	Lasagne	2.2 %
Charlie Bingham's	Moussaka	2.2 %
Charlie Bingham's	Thai Red Chicken Curry & Fragrant Rice	2.2 %
Cook	Chicken Dijon	2.2 %
Cook	Saag Paneer	2.2 %
Cook	Yellow Malaysian Fish Curry	2.2 %
Easy Bean	Indian Sambar	2.2 %
Holland's	Lancashire Hotpots	2.2 %
Kirsty's	Chicken Tikka Masala with Brown Basmati Rice	2.2 %
Linda McCartney	Asparagus & Leek Tartlets	2.2 %
Linda McCartney	Butternut Squash & Goats Cheese Tartlet	2.2 %
Linda McCartney	Cheese & Leek Plaits	2.2 %
Morrisons	Bacon & Leek Quiche	2.2 %
Morrisons	M Kitchen Fresh Ideas Chicken & Chorizo Paella	2.2 %
Morrisons	M Kitchen Fresh Ideas Thai Green Chicken Curry	2.2 %
Morrisons	The All Day Big Breakfast	2.2 %

Ready Meals – by sugar content (continued)

Brand	Label	% Sugar
Pukka-Pies	Large Stand-Up Pasty	2.2 %
Quorn	Meat Free Tikka Masala With Rice	2.2 %
Sainsbury's	Classic Lamb Dinner	2.2 %
Sainsbury's	Pub Specials Beef Lasagne	2.2 %
Sainsbury's	Pub Specials Slow Cooked Beef in Red Wine with Gratin Potatoes	2.2 %
Stagg	Homestead Minced Chili with Beans	2.2 %
Tesco	Chicken Korma	2.2 %
Tesco	Classic Italian Family Beef Lasagne	2.2 %
Tesco	Classic Italian Spinach & Ricotta Cannelloni	2.2 %
Tesco	Everyday Value Bean And Cheese Melts	2.2 %
Tesco	Finest Chicken Korma with Pilau Rice	2.2 %
Tesco	Finest Cumberland Pork Sausages & Creamy Mash	2.2 %
Tesco	Finest Slow Cooked Beef with Buttered Roast Potatoes	2.2 %
Tesco	Finest Spanish Chicken with Chorizo	2.2 %
Tesco	Healthy Living Braised Beef & Root Veg Mash	2.2 %
Tesco	Healthy Living Cheese & Bacon Crustless Quiche	2.2 %
Tesco	Indian Beef Madras and Pilau Rice	2.2 %
Tesco	Quiche Lorraine	2.2 %
Tesco	Tex Mex Spicy Beef Burrito	2.2 %
Waitrose	Love Life Spinach & Ricotta Cannelloni	2.2 %
Waitrose	Menu Beef Bourguignon	2.2 %
Waitrose	Yorkshire with Sausage and Mash	2.2 %
Weight Watchers	Bacon & Leek Crustless Quiche	2.2 %

Ready Meals - by sugar content (continued)

Brand	Label	% Sugar
Young's	Salmon Crumble	2.2 %
Tesco	Al Fresco Broad Beans & Peas with Feta	2.2 %
Tesco	Indian Saag Bhaji	2.2 %
Tesco	Takeaway No 84 Satay Chicken	2.2 %
ASDA	Beef Lasagne	2.3 %
ASDA	Chef's Special King Prawns & Chicken	2.3 %
ASDA	Chicken Curry & Rice	2.3 %
ASDA	Classic Steak & Ale with Mash	2.3 %
ASDA	Extra Special British Meatballs with Paprika Spiced Potatoes	2.3 %
ASDA	Fresh Tastes Kitchen King Prawn Linguine	2.3 %
ASDA	Fresh Tastes Kitchen Spaghetti & Meatballs	2.3 %
ASDA	Fresh Tastes Kitchen Thai Green Chicken Curry with Rice	2.3 %
ASDA	Good & Counted Chicken in Peppercorn Sauce	2.3 %
ASDA	Italian Tuna Pasta Bake	2.3 %
ASDA	Kids Chicken Casserole & Dumplings	2.3 %
ASDA	Kids Shepherd's Pie	2.3 %
ASDA	Sausage & Bean Bakes	2.3 %
Aunt Bessie's	Mini Toad in the Hole	2.3 %
Charlie Bingham's	Salmon en Croute	2.3 %
Cook	Chicken Korma	2.3 %
Georgia's Choice	Mexican Bean Bake	2.3 %
Holland's	Steak & Kidney Puddings	2.3 %
Hungry Joe's	Chicken Curry with Rice & Naan	2.3 %

Ready Meals - by sugar content (continued)

Brand	Label	% Sugar
Hungry Joe's	Joe Vs. Vindaloo with Rice & Naan	2.3 %
John West	Light Lunch French Style Tuna Salad	2.3 %
Kirsty's	Spanish Chicken with Brown Rice	2.3 %
Little Dish	Pasta Seashells with Salmon and Broccoli	2.3 %
Morrisons	M Kitchen Fresh Ideas Chicken Dinner	2.3 %
Morrisons	M Kitchen Indian Chicken Bhuna & Pilau Rice	2.3 %
Morrisons	M Kitchen Italian Meat Feast Pasta Melt	2.3 %
Morrisons	M Kitchen Tastes of Home Minced Lamb Hotpot	2.3 %
Morrisons	M Kitchen Tex Mex Chilli Con Carne & Rice	2.3 %
Morrisons	M Kitchen Tex Mex Smokin' Mexican-Style Chicken	2.3 %
Morrisons	NuMe Red Thai Chicken Curry & Rice	2.3 %
Pieminister	Shamrock Pie	2.3 %
Pukka-Pies	Microwaveable Chicken Pie	2.3 %
Pukka-Pies	Potato, Cheese & Onion Pasty	2.3 %
Quorn	Meat Free Steak Style Pie	2.3 %
Sainsbury's	Basics Chilli con Carne	2.3 %
Sainsbury's	Basics Toad in the Hole	2.3 %
Sainsbury's	Beef Stew & Dumplings Dinner	2.3 %
Sainsbury's	Classic Liver & Bacon Dinner	2.3 %
Tesco	Cheese & Onion Large Quiche	2.3 %
Tesco	Classic Italian Beef Cannelloni	2.3 %
Tesco	Everyday Value Chicken Curry with Vegetables	2.3 %
Tesco	Everyday Value Lasagne	2.3 %
Tesco	Finest Chicken Tikka Masala with Pilau Rice	2.3 %
Tesco	Finest Jalfrezi with Pilau Rice	2.3 %

Ready Meals - by sugar content (continued)

Brand	Label	% Sugar
Tesco	Finest Slow Braised Lancashire Hotpot	2.3 %
Tesco	Takeaway Thai Red & Green Chicken Curry Meal For 2	2.3 %
Tesco	Tex Mex Chicken Enchiladas	2.3 %
Tesco	Vegetable Curry	2.3 %
Toscana	Penne Beef Bolognese	2.3 %
Uncle Ben's	Rice Time Spicy Tikka Masala	2.3 %
Waitrose	Beef Casserole	2.3 %
Waitrose	Essential Bacon, Leek & Cheddar Cheese Quiche	2.3 %
Waitrose	Frozen Vegetarian Cottage Pie	2.3 %
Waitrose	Haddock in Cheese Sauce	2.3 %
Waitrose	Love Life Lasagne	2.3 %
Waitrose	Quiche Lorraine Crustless	2.3 %
Waitrose	Roast Chicken Pie	2.3 %
Waitrose	Steak Pie	2.3 %
Weight Watchers From Heinz	Salmon & Broccoli Wedge Melt	2.3 %
Young's	Fish Fillet Dinner	2.3 %
Amy's Kitchen	Gluten Free Rice Mac & Cheese	2.4 %
Amy's Kitchen	Mac & Cheese	2.4 %
Annabel Karmel	Scrumptious Chicken Tikka & Rice	2.4 %
ASDA	Bistro Chicken Filo Pastry Pie	2.4 %
ASDA	Classic Beef Stew & Dumplings	2.4 %
ASDA	Classic Corned Beef Hash	2.4 %
ASDA	Cumberland Pie for 4	2.4 %

Ready Meals - by sugar content (continued)

Brand	Label	% Sugar
ASDA	Good & Counted Beef Lasagne	2.4 %
ASDA	Good & Counted Turkey Meatballs with Mexican Herb Rice	2.4 %
ASDA	Italian Meat Feast Pasta Bake for 2	2.4 %
ASDA	Meat Feast Pasta Bake for 4	2.4 %
ASDA	Slow Cooked Steak & Gravy Pies	2.4 %
Birds Eye	Stir Your Senses Gnocchi con Gorgonzola e Spinaci	2.4 %
Charlie Bingham's	Spinach & Ricotta Cannelloni	2.4 %
Cook	Kids Fish Pie	2.4 %
Cook	Lamb Moussaka	2.4 %
Cook	Nasi Goreng	2.4 %
Cook	Thai Butternut Squash Soup	2.4 %
DS Gluten Free	Bonta d' Italia Lasagne	2.4 %
Holland's	Potato & Meat Pies	2.4 %
Levi Roots	Caribbean Curried Chicken Noodles	2.4 %
Little Dish	Mini Cheese Ravioli in Tomato & Veg Sauce	2.4 %
Little Dish	Spaghetti with Mini Meatballs	2.4 %
Low Low	Chicken Biryani	2.4 %
Morrisons	M Kitchen Fresh Ideas King Prawn Linguini	2.4 %
Morrisons	M Kitchen Italian Penne Bolognese Bake	2.4 %
Morrisons	M Kitchen Tastes of Home Minced Beef & Potatoes	2.4 %
Quorn	Meat Free Pasty	2.4 %
Sainsbury's	Basics Prawn Curry with Rice	2.4 %
Sainsbury's	Chicken Jalfrezi with Pilau Rice	2.4 %

Ready Meals - by sugar content (continued)

Brand	Label	% Sugar
Tesco	Chilli Con Carne	2.4 %
Tesco	Classic All Day Breakfast	2.4 %
Tesco	Classic Italian Roasted Vegetable Lasagne	2.4 %
Tesco	Finest Malaysian Chicken Curry and Jasmine Rice	2.4 %
Tesco	Finest Spicy Pork Meatballs Pasta	2.4 %
Tesco	Healthy Living Sweet & Sour Chicken & Rice	2.4 %
Tesco	Honey & Mustard Chicken Pasta	2.4 %
Tesco	Indian Chicken Korma & Jalfrezi Meal For 2	2.4 %
Tesco	Big Night In Chinese Chicken Curry & Egg Fried Rice	2.4 %
Tesco	Big Night Time In Beef Blackbean & Egg Fried Rice	2.4 %
Waitrose	Braised Steak, Portobello Mushroom & Red Wine Pie	2.4 %
Waitrose	Chilli con Carne with Rice	2.4 %
Waitrose	Heston Chilli Con Carne	2.4 %
Waitrose	Indian Chicken Shashlik	2.4 %
Waitrose	Liver and Bacon	2.4 %
Waitrose	Love Life Beef & Barbecue Beans	2.4 %
Waitrose	Love Life Butternut Squash Risotto	2.4 %
Waitrose	Oriental Chicken Chow Mein	2.4 %
Waitrose	Roasted Red Pepper Goats Cheese Quiche	2.4 %
Waitrose	Vintage Cheddar & Onion Small Quiche	2.4 %
Weight Watchers	Lincolnshire Sausages & Mash	2.4 %
Amy's Kitchen	Gluten Free Vegetable Lasagne	2.5 %
ASDA	Chef's Special King Prawn Korma	2.5 %

Ready Meals – by sugar content (continued)

Brand	Label	% Sugar
ASDA	Classic Favourites Minted Lamb Loin Chops	2.5 %
ASDA	Good & Balanced Turkey Meatballs & Pasta	2.5 %
ASDA	Good & Counted Beef Chilli & Wedges	2.5 %
ASDA	Indian Chicken Biryani	2.5 %
ASDA	Italian Beef Lasagne for 2	2.5 %
ASDA	Italian Spaghetti Meatballs	2.5 %
ASDA	Italian Spicy Chicken Pasta	2.5 %
ASDA	Spicy Chicken Pasta for 4	2.5 %
ASDA	Taste of America Blazin' Chicken Burrito	2.5 %
Birds Eye	Stir Your Senses Spanish Paella with Chicken and Prawn	2.5 %
Charlie Bingham's	Chicken Tikka Masala & Pilau Rice	2.5 %
Charlie Bingham's	Paella with Chicken, King Prawns & Chorizo	2.5 %
Cook	Linguine Carbonara Family Meal	2.5 %
DS Gluten Free	Quiche Lorraine	2.5 %
Kirsty's	Moroccan Vegetables with Quinoa	2.5 %
Look What We Found!	Staffordshire Chicken Thai Green Curry	2.5 %
Morrisons	Cheese & Onion Quiche	2.5 %
Morrisons	Just For Kids Fish Pie	2.5 %
Morrisons	Just for Kids Spaghetti Bolognese	2.5 %
Morrisons	M Kitchen Italian Chicken Lasagne	2.5 %
Morrisons	M Kitchen Tastes of Home Slow-Cooked Lamb Shank in a Red Wine & Rosemary Gravy	2.5 %
Morrisons	M Kitchen Tex Mex Spicy Chicken Enchilada	2.5 %

Ready Meals - by sugar content (continued)

Brand	Label	% Sugar
Morrisons	Mexican Chicken	2.5 %
Morrisons	NuMe Chilli con Carne with Rice	2.5 %
Morrisons	Signature Beef Bourguignon	2.5 %
Quorn	Meat Free Lasagne	2.5 %
Tesco	Cheese & Bacon Quiche	2.5 %
Tesco	Cheese & Onion Small Quiche	2.5 %
Tesco	Classic Italian Spaghetti & Meatballs	2.5 %
Tesco	Finest Chicken Tikka with Jewelled Rice & Lime Relish	2.5 %
Tesco	Finest Mapye Cured Bacon & Gruyere Quiche	2.5 %
Tesco	Healthy Living Chicken Arrabbiatta	2.5 %
Tesco	Indian Chicken Korma With Pilau Rice	2.5 %
Tesco	Indian Chicken Tikka & Korma Meal For 2	2.5 %
Tesco	Indian Chicken Tikka Masala Pilau Rice and Bombay Potato	2.5 %
Tesco	Italian Beef Lasagne	2.5 %
Tesco	Modern Italian Chicken Breasts with Tomato & Basil Sauce	2.5 %
Tesco	Spanish Chicken & Chorizo Paella	2.5 %
Tesco	British Classics Chicken & Bacon Pie	2.5 %
Tesco	British Classics Chicken & Mushroom Hotpot	2.5 %
The City Kitchen	Katsu Chicken Curry	2.5 %
The City Kitchen	Thai Chicken Fried Rice	2.5 %
Waitrose	Bacon, Leek & Roquefort Tart	2.5 %
Waitrose	Beef Cannelloni	2.5 %
Waitrose	Delisante Artisan Quiche Lorraine	2.5 %

Ready Meals - by sugar content (continued)

Brand	Label	% Sugar
Waitrose	Essential Cheddar Cheese & Onion Quiche	2.5 %
Waitrose	Frozen Pea & Asparagus Risotto	2.5 %
Waitrose	Indian Goan Fish Curry	2.5 %
Waitrose	Indian Vegetable Thoran	2.5 %
Waitrose	Love Life Chicken Kastu Curry & Jasmine Rice	2.5 %
Waitrose	Love Life Spicy Jerk Chicken	2.5 %
Waitrose	Spinach & Ricotta Quiche	2.5 %
Weight Watchers	Bolognese al Forno	2.5 %
Weight Watchers	Jamaican Jerk Chicken Curry with Rice	2.5 %
Weight Watchers From Heinz	Mexican Chilli	2.5 %
Young's	Low Fat Ocean Crumble	2.5 %
Amy's Kitchen	Gluten Free Vegetable Korma	2.6 %
Annabel Karmel	Tasty Chicken & Potato Pie	2.6 %
ASDA	Chef's Special Bengali Lamb Bhuna	2.6 %
ASDA	Classic Toad in the Hole with Bacon	2.6 %
ASDA	Express Meals Chinese Chicken Curry & Rice	2.6 %
ASDA	Fresh Tastes Kitchen Chicken, Char Sui Pork & Prawn Rice	2.6 %
ASDA	Good & Balanced Lemon Chicken & Wild Rice	2.6 %
ASDA	Kids Beef Chilli & Potato Wedges	2.6 %
ASDA	Smartprice Spaghetti Bolognese	2.6 %
ASDA	Toad in the Hole	2.6 %
ASDA	Vegetarian Chicken Style Casserole with Dumplings	2.6 %

Ready Meals - by sugar content (continued)

Brand	Label	% Sugar
Cook	Chilli con Carne	2.6 %
Cook	Macaroni Cheese	2.6 %
Dolmio	Bolognese Pasta Vista	2.6 %
Easy Bean	Spanish Puchero	2.6 %
Genius	Gluten Free Steak Pies	2.6 %
Heinz	Big Beef Hotpot with Chunky Veg	2.6 %
Holland's	Steak & Kidney Pies	2.6 %
Hunger Breaks	The Full Monty	2.6 %
Linda McCartney	Cheese, Leek & Red Onion Plaits	2.6 %
Morrisons	M Kitchen Indian Chicken Rogan Josh & Pilau Rice	2.6 %
Morrisons	M Kitchen Indian Tandoori Chicken & Pilau Rice	2.6 %
Morrisons	M Kitchen Italian Chicken & Ham Pasta Bake	2.6 %
Morrisons	M Kitchen Italian Three Cheese Pasta Melt	2.6 %
Morrisons	M Kitchen Oriental Chinese Chicken Curry & Egg Fried Rice	2.6 %
Morrisons	Savers Spaghetti Bolognese	2.6 %
Pieminister	Kate & Sidney Pie	2.6 %
Pieminister	Matador Pie Pot	2.6 %
Pieminister	Moo & Blue Pie	2.6 %
Princes	Chilli Con Carne	2.6 %
Quorn	Meat Free Mexican Chilli Burrito	2.6 %
Tasty Favourites	Chicken Tikka	2.6 %
Tesco	Big Night In Indian Chicken Korma & Pilau Rice	2.6 %

Ready Meals - by sugar content (continued)

Brand	Label	% Sugar
Tesco	Cheese & Onion Quiche	2.6 %
Tesco	Classic Italian Tomato & Mozzarella Pasta Bake	2.6 %
Tesco	Finest Mapye Cured Bacon & Gruyere Small Quiche	2.6 %
Tesco	Finest Red Thai Duck Noodles	2.6 %
Tesco	Indian Chicken Jalfrezi and Pilau Rice	2.6 %
Tesco	Indian Chicken Tikka Masala & Lamb Rogan Josh Meal For 2	2.6 %
Tesco	Indian Lamb Rogan Josh and Pilau Rice	2.6 %
Tesco	Modern Italian Fajita Chicken Pasta	2.6 %
Waitrose	Beef Lasagne	2.6 %
Waitrose	Chicken Enchiladas	2.6 %
Waitrose	Love Life Chicken Korma with Pilau Rice	2.6 %
Waitrose	Love Life Tomato & Rosemary Chicken	2.6 %
Waitrose	Mushroom & Spinach Filo Parcel	2.6 %
Waitrose	Roast Beef Dinner	2.6 %
Waitrose	Rosemary Chicken Penne	2.6 %
Waitrose	Vintage Cheddar & Onion Quiche	2.6 %
Weight Watchers	Hunters Chicken with Brown & Wild Rice	2.6 %
Weight Watchers From Heinz	Chicken Hotpot	2.6 %
Young's	Salmon Fillet Dinner	2.6 %
Tesco	Indian Prawn Masala and Pilau Rice	2.6 %
Amy's Kitchen	Gluten Free Vegetable Lasagne	2.7 %
ASDA	Chicken Tandoori Masala with Pilau Rice	2.7 %

Ready Meals - by sugar content (continued)

Brand	Label	% Sugar
ASDA	Extra Special West Country Beef Brisket with Theakstons Ale	2.7 %
ASDA	Family Carbonara	2.7 %
ASDA	Good & Balanced Oriental Pork with Rice & Lentils	2.7 %
ASDA	Italian Beef Lasagne	2.7 %
ASDA	Taste of America Cheesy Nacho Chicken Pasta Melt	2.7 %
ASDA	Taste of America Inferno Sloppy Joe	2.7 %
ASDA	Taste of America Stacked Chicken & Pepperoni Spicy Pasta Melt	2.7 %
Cook	Cottage Pie	2.7 %
Cook	Shepherd's Pie	2.7 %
Holland's	Minced Beef & Onion Pies	2.7 %
John West	Light Lunch Mexican Style Tuna Salad	2.7 %
Linda McCartney	Lentil & Vegetable Cottage Pie	2.7 %
Little Dish	Mild Chicken Curry with Rice	2.7 %
Little Dish	Pork and Apple Bites with Beans	2.7 %
Morrisons	M Kitchen Indian Chicken Jalfrezi & Pilau Rice	2.7 %
Morrisons	M Kitchen Indian Takeaway Aloo Gobi Saag	2.7 %
Morrisons	M Kitchen Indian Takeaway Korma & Tikka Masala Meal for 2	2.7 %
Morrisons	M Kitchen Tex Mex Blazin' Chicken Burrito	2.7 %
Pieminister	Moo & Brew Pie Pot	2.7 %
Pooles	Minced Beef & Onion Pies	2.7 %
Pukka-Pies	Large Chicken & Mushroom Pie	2.7 %
Sainsbury's	Chicken Korma with Rice	2.7 %

Ready Meals - by sugar content (continued)

Brand	Label	% Sugar
Sainsbury's	Chip Shop Chicken Curry	2.7 %
Sainsbury's	Italian Beef Lasagne	2.7 %
Tesco	Al Fresco King Prawn & Orzo Pasta	2.7 %
Tesco	Classic Italian Chicken Lasagne	2.7 %
Tesco	Everyday Value Chicken Korma And Rice	2.7 %
Tesco	Family Favourites Chicken & Tomato Pasta Bake	2.7 %
Tesco	Finest Creamy Fish Pie	2.7 %
Tesco	Healthy Living Chicken Tikka Masala & Rice	2.7 %
Tesco	Healthy Living Sausage & Root Veg Mash	2.7 %
Tesco	Indian Chicken Tikka Masala and Pilau Rice	2.7 %
Tesco	Modern Italian Chicken Arrabbiata Pasta	2.7 %
Tesco	Modern Italian Pepperoni Pasta Bake	2.7 %
Tesco	Takeaway Indian Chicken Korma with Pilau Rice & Naan Bread	2.7 %
Waitrose	Chicken Arrabiata	2.7 %
Waitrose	Frozen Mini Lasagne	2.7 %
Waitrose	Frozen Vegetarian Chestnuts & Mushroom Grills	2.7 %
Waitrose	Menu Beef Lasagne	2.7 %
Weight Watchers	Szechuan Chicken with Rice	2.7 %
Levi Roots	Caribbean Hot Chilli Beef with Seasoned Rice	2.7 %
Uncle Ben's	Rice Time Medium Curry	2.7 %
Tesco	Oriental Kung Po Chicken with Egg Fried Rice	2.8 %
Uncle Ben's	Rice Time Mexican Chilli	2.8 %
Amoy	Nasi Goreng Meal Kit	2.8 %
Amy's Kitchen	All American Veggie Burger	2.8 %

Ready Meals - by sugar content (continued)

Brand	Label	% Sugar
Amy's Kitchen	Gluten Free Indian Mattar Paneer	2.8 %
Amy's Kitchen	Gluten Free Manhattan Veggie Burger	2.8 %
Annabel Karmel	Scrummy Salmon & Cod Fish Pie	2.8 %
ASDA	Extra Special Tandoori Chicken with Chickpea Rice	2.8 %
ASDA	Extra Special West Country Beef Lasagne for 1	2.8 %
ASDA	Fresh Tastes Kitchen Chicken Pasta in White Wine Sauce	2.8 %
ASDA	Good & Counted Chicken & King Prawn Paella	2.8 %
ASDA	Italian Chicken & Tomato Pasta Melt for 2	2.8 %
ASDA	Italian Spinach & Ricotta Cannelloni	2.8 %
ASDA	Italian Tomato & Mozzarella Pasta Bake	2.8 %
ASDA	Kids Cheese Ravioli	2.8 %
ASDA	Smartprice Lasagne	2.8 %
ASDA	Smartprice Minced Beef & Onion Pies	2.8 %
ASDA	Taste of America Loaded Hot Dog Style Chilli Bake	2.8 %
ASDA	Taste of America Mouth-Watering Beefy Burritos	2.8 %
ASDA	Tomato & Mozzarella Pasta Bake for 4	2.8 %
Birds Eye	Stir Your Senses Penne all Arrabbiata con Pollo	2.8 %
Cook	Chicken Noodle Laksa For 2	2.8 %
Cook	Lamb Hotpot	2.8 %
Genius	Gluten Free Vegetable Curry Pies	2.8 %
Hungry Joe's	Cajun Chicken & Spicy Rice	2.8 %
Hungry Joe's	Mighty Meatball Pasta Feast	2.8 %

Ready Meals – by sugar content (continued)

Brand	Label	% Sugar
Linda McCartney	Vegetarian Sausage & Vegetable Hot Pot	2.8 %
Little Dish	British Lamb Hotpot	2.8 %
Little Dish	Classic Beef Lasagne	2.8 %
Little Dish	Cottage Pie with Seven Veg	2.8 %
Look What We Found!	Staffordshire Chicken Thai Red Curry	2.8 %
Look What We Found!	Yorkshire Pork Sausage Casserole	2.8 %
Morrisons	M Kitchen Italian King Prawn Linguine	2.8 %
Morrisons	M Kitchen Italian Lasagne	2.8 %
Morrisons	M Kitchen Italian Vegetable Lasagne	2.8 %
Morrisons	NuMe Lasagne	2.8 %
Morrisons	Savers Beef Lasagne	2.8 %
Morrisons	Signature Aberdeen Angus Lasagne	2.8 %
Princes	Mexican Tuna Salad	2.8 %
Sainsbury's	Butter Chicken with Rice	2.8 %
Sainsbury's	Vegetarian Vegetable Lasagne	2.8 %
Tesco	Chicken Jalfrezi	2.8 %
Tesco	Chinese Beef & Black Bean Sauce	2.8 %
Tesco	Family Favourites Lasagne	2.8 %
Tesco	Finest Beef Madras with Pilau Rice	2.8 %
Tesco	Finest Hot Piri Piri Chicken and Rice	2.8 %
Tesco	Indian Chicken Tikka Masala & Jalfrezi Meal For 2	2.8 %
Tesco	Thai Chicken Red Curry with Jasmine Rice	2.8 %
The City Kitchen	King Prawn Red Thai Curry	2.8 %

Ready Meals - by sugar content (continued)

Brand	Label	% Sugar
Waitrose	Leek Gratin	2.8 %
Waitrose	Love Life Beef & Pork Meatballs with Spaghetti	2.8 %
Waitrose	Love Life Chicken & Prawn Paella	2.8 %
Waitrose	Menu Beef Casserole	2.8 %
Young's	Mariner's Pie	2.8 %
The City Kitchen	Indonesian Pulled Pork & Mushroom Noodles	2.9 %
Annabel Karmel	Delicious Beef Cottage Pie	2.9 %
ASDA	Beef Lasagne for 4	2.9 %
ASDA	Chicken & Mushrooms	2.9 %
ASDA	Classic Moussaka	2.9 %
ASDA	Extra Special West Country Beef Lasagne for 2	2.9 %
ASDA	Fresh Tastes Kitchen Chicken Tikka Masala & Rice	2.9 %
ASDA	Fresh Tastes Kitchen Malaysian Chicken Curry	2.9 %
ASDA	Fresh Tastes Kitchen Red Thai King Prawn Curry & Noodles	2.9 %
ASDA	Good & Balanced Italian Chicken & Tomato Wholemeal Pasta	2.9 %
ASDA	Good & Counted Beef Lasagne	2.9 %
ASDA	Kids Cheese & Creamy Tomato Pasta	2.9 %
ASDA	Kids Roast Chicken & Gravy Pie	2.9 %
ASDA	Pub Classics Chicken Jalfrezi with Lemon Rice	2.9 %
ASDA	Sizzler Fajita Chicken for 2	2.9 %
ASDA	Smartprice Bolognese Pasta Bake	2.9 %
ASDA	Vegetable Chow Mein	2.9 %
Cook	Red Thai Chicken Curry	2.9 %

Ready Meals - by sugar content (continued)

Brand	Label	% Sugar
Dolmio	Tomato & Basil Pasta Vista	2.9 %
Georgia's Choice	Beef Lasagne	2.9 %
Gino's	Deep Pan Pepperoni Pizza	2.9 %
Holland's	Pub Classics Peppered Steak Pie	2.9 %
Low Low	Chicken & Chorizo Paella	2.9 %
Morrisons	M Kitchen Fresh Ideas Beef in Ale	2.9 %
Morrisons	M Kitchen Fresh Ideas Moroccan Chicken	2.9 %
Morrisons	M Kitchen Tex Mex Sizzlin' Salsa Chicken	2.9 %
Morrisons	M Kitchen Vegetarian Paneer Jalfrezi with Pilau Rice	2.9 %
Morrisons	NuMe Quiche Lorraine	2.9 %
Quorn	Meat Free Piri Piri & Rice	2.9 %
Sainsbury's	Chickpea & Chorizo Stew	2.9 %
Sainsbury's	Vegetable Pies	2.9 %
Tesco	Big Night In Indian Vegetable Balti & Pilau Rice	2.9 %
Tesco	Classic Italian Meatball Pasta Bake	2.9 %
Tesco	Everyday Value Chicken Tikka And Rice	2.9 %
Tesco	Finest Bourbon Pulled Beef & Sweet Onion Mash	2.9 %
The City Kitchen	Chilli Moonshine Beef	2.9 %
Waitrose	Frozen Vegetarian Goats Cheese & Spinach Slices	2.9 %
Waitrose	Indian Aloo Gobi Saag	2.9 %
Waitrose	Love Life Lamb Moussaka	2.9 %
Waitrose	Love Life Roasted Vegetable Lasagne	2.9 %
Amy's Kitchen	Gluten Free Thai Red Curry	3.0 %

Ready Meals - by sugar content (continued)

Brand	Label	% Sugar
Annabel Karmel	Veggie Pasta Bake with Butternut Squash	3.0 %
ASDA	Classic All Day Breakfast	3.0 %
ASDA	Extra Special Venison Casserole with Sloe Gin & Potato	3.0 %
ASDA	Fresh Tastes Kitchen Piri Piri Chicken & Rice	3.0 %
ASDA	Fresh Tastes Kitchen Red Thai Chicken Curry & Rice	3.0 %
ASDA	Fresh Tastes Kitchen Sweet Chilli Beef Noodles	3.0 %
ASDA	Good & Balanced Moroccan Lamb Meatballs with Cous Cous	3.0 %
ASDA	Good & Balanced Tandoori Chicken with Basmati Rice	3.0 %
ASDA	Good & Counted Ham Hock with Root Mash	3.0 %
ASDA	Good & Counted Spinach & Ricotta Cannelloni	3.0 %
ASDA	Italian Sausage Pasta Bake	3.0 %
ASDA	Italian Sausage Pasta Bake for 2	3.0 %
ASDA	Sausage Pasta Bake for 4	3.0 %
ASDA	Vegetarian Pepper & Courgette Lasagne	3.0 %
ASDA	Vegetarian Sweet Potato & Mozzarella Bakes	3.0 %
Baxters	Malaysian Inspired Chicken Laksa	3.0 %
Birds Eye	Mediterranean Vegetable Penne Pasta	3.0 %
Birds Eye	Steamfresh Mediterranean Vegetable Pasta	3.0 %
Birds Eye	Traditional Beef with Homestyle Gravy	3.0 %
Cook	Beef Bolognese Pasta Bake Family Meal	3.0 %
Cook	Japanese Salmon	3.0 %
Cook	Keralan Prawn Curry	3.0 %
Easy Bean	French Cuisinés	3.0 %

Ready Meals - by sugar content (continued)

Brand	Label	% Sugar
Fray Bentos	Hunger Burster Meatballs & Pasta	3.0 %
Giovanni Rana	Lasagne Bolognese	3.0 %
Little Dish	Alphabet Pasta Bolognese	3.0 %
Low Low	Chicken Tomato & Basil Pasta	3.0 %
Morrisons	M Kitchen Fresh Ideas Chicken en Croute	3.0 %
Morrisons	M Kitchen Indian Chicken Tikka Masala & Pilau Rice	3.0 %
Our Little Secret	Flavoursome Curried Chicken Rice	3.0 %
Quorn	Meat Free Chicken Style & Leek Pie	3.0 %
Quorn	Meat Free Chilli & Wedges	3.0 %
Sainsbury's	Basics Spaghetti Bolognese	3.0 %
Sainsbury's	Beef Bolognese	3.0 %
Sharwood's	Chicken Tikka Masala with Rice	3.0 %
Stagg	Classic Chili con Carne	3.0 %
Stagg	Dynamite Hot Chili con Carne	3.0 %
Stagg	Silverado Beef Chili con Carne	3.0 %
Tesco	Cheese & Tomato Quiche	3.0 %
Tesco	Classic Italian Sausage Pasta Bake	3.0 %
Tesco	Healthy Living Broccoli & Tomato Crustless Quiche	3.0 %
Tesco	Sweet Potato & Goat's Cheese Lattice Pie	3.0 %
Tesco	Al Fresco Spanish Pork & Chorizo Meatballs in Tomato Sauce	3.0 %
Tesco	Oriental Chinese Chicken Curry with Egg Fried Rice	3.0 %
Tesco	Oriental Meal For 2 Menu C	3.0 %

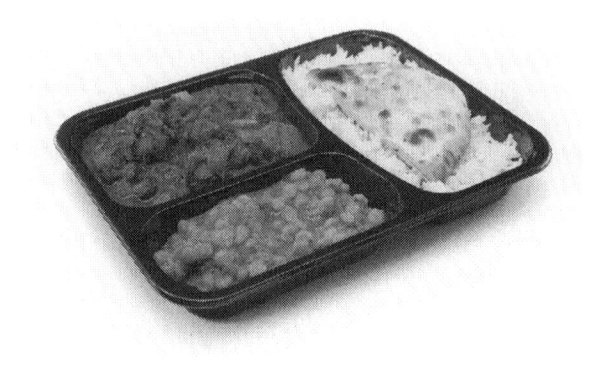

Ready Meals - by sugar content (continued)

Brand	Label	% Sugar
Toscana	Penne Tomato & Basil	3.0 %
Toscana	Penne Tomato & Chilli	3.0 %
Waitrose	Four Cheese Ravioli	3.0 %
Waitrose	Frozen Vegetarian Lasagne	3.0 %
Waitrose	Indian Lamb Kofta Curry	3.0 %

Ready Meals - by brand

Brand	Label	% Sugar
Amoy	Malaysian Laksa Meal Kit	0.7 %
	Thai Red Curry Meal Kit	0.7 %
	Thai Green Curry Meal Kit	0.8 %
	Nasi Goreng Meal Kit	2.8 %
Amy's Kitchen	Gluten Dairy Free Rice Mac & Cheeze	0.0 %
	Cheddar, Rice & Bean Burrito	0.6 %
	Bean & Rice Burrito	1.2 %
	Gluten Free Black Bean & Vegetable Enchilada	1.5 %
	Gluten Free Cheese Enchilada	1.6 %
	Gluten Free Bean & Rice Burrito	1.9 %
	Gluten Free Cheddar, Rice & Bean Burrito	1.9 %
	Vegetable Lasagne	1.9 %
	Gluten Free Broccoli & Cheddar Bake	2.1 %
	Gluten Free Mexican Tortilla Bake	2.2 %
	Gluten Free Rice Mac & Cheese	2.4 %
	Mac & Cheese	2.4 %
	Gluten Free Vegetable Lasagne	2.5 %
	Gluten Free Vegetable Korma	2.6 %
	Gluten Free Vegetable Lasagne	2.7 %
	All American Veggie Burger	2.8 %
	Gluten Free Indian Mattar Paneer	2.8 %
	Gluten Free Manhattan Veggie Burger	2.8 %
	Gluten Free Thai Red Curry	3.0 %
	Scrummy Chicken & Rice	2.2 %
	Scrumptious Chicken Tikka & Rice	2.4 %

Ready Meals - by brand (continued)

Brand	Label	% Sugar
Annabel Karmel	Tasty Chicken & Potato Pie	2.6 %
	Scrummy Salmon & Cod Fish Pie	2.8 %
	Delicious Beef Cottage Pie	2.9 %
	Veggie Pasta Bake with Butternut Squash	3.0 %
ASDA	Chicken & Bacon Puff Pastry Lattice	0.1 %
	Chicken & Ham Bakes	0.1 %
	Classic Cottage Pie	0.1 %
	Classic Cumberland Pie	0.1 %
	Classic Fish Pie	0.1 %
	Classic Roast Beef Dinner in a Giant Yorkshire	0.1 %
	Classic Roast Chicken Dinner	0.1 %
	Extra Special Luxury Fish Pie	0.1 %
	Family Chicken & Vegetable Puff Pastry Pie	0.1 %
	Classic Favourites Chicken Wrapped in Bacon	0.2 %
	Classic Favourites Ham & Mushroom Chicken	0.2 %
	Classic Gammon Dinner	0.2 %
	Classic Haddock & Chips	0.2 %
	Italian Chicken & Pesto Penne Pasta	0.2 %
	Steak & Kidney Puff Pastry Pie	0.2 %
	Tiger Cheese & Onion Puff Pastry Pie	0.2 %
	Chicken Tikka Masala & Jalfrezi for 2	0.3 %
	Classic Favourites Chicken Kiev	0.3 %
	Classic Roast Beef Dinner	0.3 %
	Family Minced Steak & Onion Puff Pastry Pie	0.3 %
	Kids Chicken Tikka Masala	0.3 %

Ready Meals - by brand (continued)

Brand	Label	% Sugar
ASDA	Steak & Ale Puff Pastry Pie	0.3 %
	Classic Chicken Breasts in Red Wine Sauce for 2	0.4 %
	Classic Favourites Cod Pie	0.4 %
	Classic Favourites Gammon & Cheese	0.4 %
	Classic Roast Pork Dinner with Crackling	0.4 %
	Family Steak & Potato Puff Pastry Pie	0.4 %
	Steak & Stilton Puff Pastry Pie	0.4 %
	Classic Favourites Cod with Cheese Sauce	0.5 %
	Classic Ham Hock in Parsley Sauce & Mash	0.5 %
	Good & Counted Chicken Enchiladas	0.5 %
	Spaghetti Bolognese	0.5 %
	World Favourites Lime & Coriander Chicken	0.5 %
	Chicken & Gravy Shortcrust Pastry Pie	0.6 %
	Classic Hunter's Chicken	0.6 %
	Classic Roast Chicken Dinner in a Giant Yorkshire	0.6 %
	Cottage Pie	0.6 %
	Indian Hot & Spicy Chicken Tikka Masala with Palau Rice & Bombay Potatoes	0.6 %
	Italian Chicken & Mushroom Risotto	0.6 %
	Kids Roast Chicken Dinner	0.6 %
	Steak & Gravy Puff Pastry Pie	0.6 %
	Steak & Gravy Shortcrust Pastry Pie	0.6 %
	Chicken & Gravy Large Puff Pastry Pie	0.7 %
	Chicken Shortcrust Pie	0.7 %
	Classic Chicken Bacon And Leek Pie for 2	0.7 %
	Family Favourites Cottage Pie	0.7 %

Ready Meals - by brand (continued)

Brand	Label	% Sugar
ASDA	Minced Steak & Onion Puff Pastry Pie	0.7 %
	Pork Sausage & Onion Puff Pastry Plait	0.7 %
	Steak & Gravy Large Shortcrust Pastry Pie	0.7 %
	Vegetarian Creamy Potato, Cheese & Onion Pie	0.7 %
	Bistro Ultimate Steak Pie	0.8 %
	Chicken & Mushroom with Egg Fried Rice	0.8 %
	Classic Favourites Peppercorn Chicken	0.8 %
	Classic Sausage & Mash	0.8 %
	Extra Special Salmon en Croute	0.8 %
	Family Size Deep Filled Chicken & Vegetable Pie	0.8 %
	Italian Chicken & Pesto Pasta Melt	0.8 %
	Italian Ham, Mushroom & Mascarpone Pasta Melt for 2	0.8 %
	Minced Beef & Onion Shortcrust Pie	0.8 %
	Prawn Curry & Rice	0.8 %
	Roast Chicken Dinner	0.8 %
	Smartprice Sausage and Mash	0.8 %
	Steak Pie	0.8 %
	Bistro Pork, Bramley Apple & Cider Pie	0.9 %
	Chicken & White Wine Puff Pastry Pie	0.9 %
	Chicken Tikka Masala with Pilau Rice	0.9 %
	Classic Chicken, Leek & Bacon Pie	0.9 %
	Extra Special King Prawn Linguine	0.9 %
	Extra Special Spiced Lamb with Bombay Potatoes & Tarka Dahl	0.9 %
	Indian Creamy Butter Chicken Masal with Pilau Rice & Bhajis	0.9 %

Ready Meals - by brand (continued)

Brand	Label	% Sugar
ASDA	Italian Spaghetti Carbonara	0.9 %
	Pub Classics Sausage & Mash	0.9 %
	Smartprice Fish Pie	0.9 %
	Steak & Ale Large Puff Pastry Pie	0.9 %
	Steak & Kidney Puff Pastry Pie	0.9 %
	Steak & Onion Puff Pastry Lattice	0.9 %
	Steak & Red Wine Large Puff Pastry Pie	0.9 %
	Deep Filled Slow-Cooked Steak & Gravy Pie	1.0 %
	Extra Special Slow-Cooked Beef Stroganoff	1.0 %
	Extra Special West Country Beef Cottage Pie with Gentleman Jack Ale	1.0 %
	Kids Macaroni Cheese with Veg	1.0 %
	Peppered Steak Puff Pastry Pie	1.0 %
	Chicken & Gravy Large Shortcrust Pastry Pie	1.1 %
	Chicken Biryani for 2	1.1 %
	Classic Liver & Bacon with Colcannon Mash	1.1 %
	Classic Shepherds Pie	1.1 %
	Classic Shepherd's Pie	1.1 %
	Extra Special King Prawn Curry with Coconut & Mustard Rice	1.1 %
	Good & Balanced Moroccan Chicken with Bulgur Wheat	1.1 %
	Indian Chicken Balti with Pilau Rice	1.1 %
	Indian Chicken Bhuna with Pilau Rice	1.1 %
	Italian Chicken & Bacon Pasta Bake	1.1 %
	Italian Chicken & Bacon Pasta Bake	1.1 %
	Italian Macaroni Cheese	1.1 %

Ready Meals - by brand (continued)

Brand	Label	% Sugar
ASDA	Chicken Singapore Noodles	1.2 %
	Classic Beef in Peppercorn Sauce	1.2 %
	Classic Favourites Chicken En Croute	1.2 %
	Classic Roast Chicken with Peppercorn Sauce	1.2 %
	Extra Special Beer Battered Cod with Chunky Chips & Pea Puree	1.2 %
	Extra Special Shepherd's Pie	1.2 %
	Good & Counted Chinese Chicken Curry & Rice	1.2 %
	Mini Classics Lamb Hotpot	1.2 %
	Bistro Ultimate Steak & Ale Pie	1.3 %
	Chicken Filled Giant Yorkshire Pudding	1.3 %
	Chicken in Blackbean Sauce	1.3 %
	Classic Chicken Breasts in Peppercorn Sauce for 2	1.3 %
	Classic Favourites Chicken Mini Roasts	1.3 %
	Classic Haddock Mornay	1.3 %
	Classic Minced Beef & Dumplings for 2	1.3 %
	Classic Minced Beef Hot Pot	1.3 %
	Classic Minced Beef Hotpot for 4	1.3 %
	Fresh Tastes Kitchen Chicken & Mushroom Risotto	1.3 %
	Minced Beef & Dumplings for 4	1.3 %
	Minced Beef Hotpot	1.3 %
	Singapore Chicken Noodles	1.3 %
	Smartprice Minced Beef & Dumplings	1.3 %
	Vegetarian Mushroom Risotto	1.3 %
	Cheese & Onion Pie	1.4 %
	Chinese Chicken Chop Suey with Egg Fried Rice	1.4 %

Ready Meals - by brand (continued)

Brand	Label	% Sugar
ASDA	Classic Chicken Hotpot	1.4 %
	Classic Chicken, Leek & Bacon Bake	1.4 %
	Classic Minced Beef Hot Pot for 2	1.4 %
	Good & Counted Chicken Tikka Masala with Pilau Rice	1.4 %
	Good & Counted Cottage Pie	1.4 %
	Mini Classics Chicken Hotpot	1.4 %
	Roast Beef Dinner	1.4 %
	Sausage & Onion Shortcrust Pie	1.4 %
	Vegetarian Chilli Burrito	1.4 %
	Chef's Special Singapore Noodles	1.5 %
	Chicken Curry Pies	1.5 %
	Classic Chicken, Leek & Bacon Bake for 2	1.5 %
	Classic Sausages & Mash	1.5 %
	Good & Counted Fish Pie	1.5 %
	Italian Beef Bolognese Pasta Bake	1.5 %
	Italian Ham & Mushroom Tagliatelle	1.5 %
	Pub Classics Peppercorn Chicken with Sautéed Potatoes	1.5 %
	Smart Price Minced Beef & Onion Pies	1.5 %
	Smartprice Chicken Curry & Rice	1.5 %
	Smartprice Spaghetti Carbonara	1.5 %
	Vegetarian Spicy Three Bean Enchiladas	1.5 %
	Chicken & Asparagus Large Puff Pastry Pie	1.6 %
	Chicken Madras with Pilau Rice	1.6 %
	Extra Special Lamb Hotpot with Wainwright Ale	1.6 %

Ready Meals - by brand (continued)

Brand	Label	% Sugar
ASDA	Family Size Deep Filled Slow-Cooked Steak & Gravy Pie	1.6 %
	Fresh Tastes Kitchen Chicken & Bacon Carbonara	1.6 %
	Good & Balanced Chicken Tikka & Aubergine Dahl	1.6 %
	Good & Balanced Seafood Paella	1.6 %
	Good & Counted Tuna Pasta Bake	1.6 %
	Italian Chicken & Mushroom Tagliatelle	1.6 %
	Italian Spaghetti Carbonara	1.6 %
	Mini Classics Fish Pie	1.6 %
	Pasta Carbonara for 4	1.6 %
	Steak & Gravy Large Puff Pastry Pie	1.6 %
	Steak & Potato Puff Pastry Plait	1.6 %
	Taste of America Homestyle Beefy Chilli & Rice	1.6 %
	Taste of America Mighty Fine Blue Cheese Mac & Bacon	1.6 %
	Chef's Special Kerala Beef & Black Pepper Sauce	1.7 %
	Chicken Korma with Pilau Rice	1.7 %
	Chinese Chicken Curry with Egg Fried Rice	1.7 %
	Extra Special Lamb Moussaka for 2	1.7 %
	Fresh Tastes Kitchen Chinese Chicken Curry & Rice	1.7 %
	Indian Scorching Hot Chicken Vindaloo with Pilau Rice	1.7 %
	Italian Spaghetti Bolognese	1.7 %
	Italian Three Cheese & Tomato Pasta Bake	1.7 %
	Italian Three Cheese & Tomato Pasta Bake for 2	1.7 %
	Mexican Chilli & Rice for 4	1.7 %
	Pub Classics Boozy Beef Pie	1.7 %

Ready Meals - by brand (continued)

Brand	Label	% Sugar
ASDA	Smartprice Cottage Pie	1.7 %
	Vegetable & Cheese Pies	1.7 %
	Chinese Chicken Chow Mein	1.8 %
	Chinese Chicken in Blackbean Sauce	1.8 %
	Classic Liver & Bacon with Mashed	1.8 %
	Express Meals Chicken Paella	1.8 %
	Fresh Tastes Kitchen Chicken & Mushroom Stroganoff	1.8 %
	Italian Beef Bolognese Pasta Bake for 2	1.8 %
	Italian King Prawn Linguine	1.8 %
	Kids Bangers & Mash	1.8 %
	Kids Lamb Hotpot	1.8 %
	Pub Classics Gammon & Mash	1.8 %
	Salmon & Broccoli Puff Pastry Lattice	1.8 %
	Smartprice Macaroni Cheese	1.8 %
	Taste of America Finger Lickin' Southern Fried Chicken & Spicy Wedges	1.8 %
	Taste of America Mucho Gusto Meatballs & Herby Rice	1.8 %
	Cheese & Onion Bakes	1.9 %
	Chicken & Mushroom Pies	1.9 %
	Chicken Hotpot	1.9 %
	Chicken in Red Wine with Creamy Garlic Potatoes	1.9 %
	Classic Beef Goulash & Dumplings	1.9 %
	Deep Filled Roast Chicken Pie	1.9 %
	Extra Special Four Cheese Macaroni	1.9 %
	Extra Special Lamb Moussaka for 1	1.9 %

Ready Meals - by brand (continued)

Brand	Label	% Sugar
ASDA	Fish Pie	1.9 %
	Good & Counted Tomato & Mascarpone Pasta Bake	1.9 %
	Italian Pepperoni Pasta Bake	1.9 %
	Mini Classics Beef Stew & Dumpling	1.9 %
	Chicken Curried Rice	2.0 %
	Chicken Jalfrezi with Pilau Rice	2.0 %
	Chicken Korma	2.0 %
	Extra Special Chicken, Chorizo & King Prawn Paella	2.0 %
	Extra Special Spicy Chilli Steak & Rice	2.0 %
	Fresh Tastes Kitchen Chicken Chow Mein	2.0 %
	Fresh Tastes Kitchen Ham Hock with Potatoes	2.0 %
	Good & Counted Cottage Pie	2.0 %
	Italian Beef Cannelloni	2.0 %
	Italian Chicken Tagliatelle	2.0 %
	Italian Meatball Pasta Bake for 2	2.0 %
	Kids Spaghetti Bolognese	2.0 %
	Chicken Casserole for 4	2.1 %
	Chicken Chow Mein	2.1 %
	Classic All Day Breakfast	2.1 %
	Classic Chicken Pie & Mash	2.1 %
	Extra Special Spaghetti Bolognese	2.1 %
	Extra Special West Country Beef Bourguignon	2.1 %
	Family Favourites Beef Lasagne	2.1 %
	Fresh Tastes Kitchen Chicken & King Prawn Paella	2.1 %
	Fresh Tastes Kitchen Pad Thai Chicken Noodles	2.1 %
	Fresh Tastes Kitchen Spicy Chicken & Chorizo Pasta	2.1 %

Ready Meals - by brand (continued)

Brand	Label	% Sugar
ASDA	Good & Counted Beef Chilli & Rice	2.1 %
	Good & Counted Chicken Hotpot	2.1 %
	Good & Counted Chicken Nacho Bake with Potato Wedges	2.1 %
	Italian Chicken Lasagne	2.1 %
	Kids Chicken & Butternut Squash Risotto	2.1 %
	Kids Pasta Bolognese	2.1 %
	Kids Spaghetti & Meatballs	2.1 %
	Loaded Spicy Pepperoni Pasta Bake Meal for 2	2.1 %
	Mini Classics Chilli & Rice	2.1 %
	Smartprice Lasagne for 4	2.1 %
	Taste of America Kickin' Chicken Enchiladas	2.1 %
	Chicken & Vegetable Pies	2.2 %
	Chicken Chow Mein	2.2 %
	Chicken Curry Bakes	2.2 %
	Classic Beef & Ale Stew with Dumplings	2.2 %
	Fresh Tastes Kitchen Roast Chicken Dinner	2.2 %
	Good & Balanced Chicken & Roasted Butternut Squash Pasta	2.2 %
	Good & Counted Chicken Chow Mein	2.2 %
	Indian Chicken Tikka Masala with Pilau Rice	2.2 %
	Italian Chilli Beef Pasta Bake for 2	2.2 %
	Kids Cottage Pie	2.2 %
	Kids Fish Pie	2.2 %
	Beef Lasagne	2.3 %
	Chef's Special King Prawns & Chicken	2.3 %
	Chicken Curry & Rice	2.3 %

Ready Meals - by brand (continued)

Brand	Label	% Sugar
ASDA	Classic Steak & Ale with Mash	2.3 %
	Extra Special British Meatballs with Paprika Spiced Potatoes	2.3 %
	Fresh Tastes Kitchen King Prawn Linguine	2.3 %
	Fresh Tastes Kitchen Spaghetti & Meatballs	2.3 %
	Fresh Tastes Kitchen Thai Green Chicken Curry with Rice	2.3 %
	Good & Counted Chicken in Peppercorn Sauce	2.3 %
	Italian Tuna Pasta Bake	2.3 %
	Kids Chicken Casserole & Dumplings	2.3 %
	Kids Shepherd's Pie	2.3 %
	Sausage & Bean Bakes	2.3 %
	Bistro Chicken Filo Pastry Pie	2.4 %
	Classic Beef Stew & Dumplings	2.4 %
	Classic Corned Beef Hash	2.4 %
	Cumberland Pie for 4	2.4 %
	Good & Counted Beef Lasagne	2.4 %
	Good & Counted Turkey Meatballs with Mexican Herb Rice	2.4 %
	Italian Meat Feast Pasta Bake for 2	2.4 %
	Meat Feast Pasta Bake for 4	2.4 %
	Slow Cooked Steak & Gravy Pies	2.4 %
	Chef's Special King Prawn Korma	2.5 %
	Classic Favourites Minted Lamb Loin Chops	2.5 %
	Good & Balanced Turkey Meatballs & Pasta	2.5 %
	Good & Counted Beef Chilli & Wedges	2.5 %
	Indian Chicken Biryani	2.5 %

Ready Meals - by brand (continued)

Brand	Label	% Sugar
ASDA	Italian Beef Lasagne for 2	2.5 %
	Italian Spaghetti Meatballs	2.5 %
	Italian Spicy Chicken Pasta	2.5 %
	Spicy Chicken Pasta for 4	2.5 %
	Taste of America Blazin' Chicken Burrito	2.5 %
	Chef's Special Bengali Lamb Bhuna	2.6 %
	Classic Toad in the Hole with Bacon	2.6 %
	Express Meals Chinese Chicken Curry & Rice	2.6 %
	Fresh Tastes Kitchen Chicken, Char Sui Pork & Prawn Rice	2.6 %
	Good & Balanced Lemon Chicken & Wild Rice	2.6 %
	Kids Beef Chilli & Potato Wedges	2.6 %
	Smartprice Spaghetti Bolognese	2.6 %
	Toad in the Hole	2.6 %
	Vegetarian Chicken Style Casserole with Dumplings	2.6 %
	Chicken Tandoori Masala with Pilau Rice	2.7 %
	Extra Special West Country Beef Brisket with Theakstons Ale	2.7 %
	Family Carbonara	2.7 %
	Good & Balanced Oriental Pork with Rice & Lentils	2.7 %
	Italian Beef Lasagne	2.7 %
	Taste of America Cheesy Nacho Chicken Pasta Melt	2.7 %
	Taste of America Inferno Sloppy Joe	2.7 %
	Taste of America Stacked Chicken & Pepperoni Spicy Pasta Melt	2.7 %
	Extra Special Tandoori Chicken with Chickpea Rice	2.8 %
	Extra Special West Country Beef Lasagne for 1	2.8 %

Ready Meals - by brand (continued)

Brand	Label	% Sugar
ASDA	Fresh Tastes Kitchen Chicken Pasta in White Wine Sauce	2.8 %
	Good & Counted Chicken & King Prawn Paella	2.8 %
	Italian Chicken & Tomato Pasta Melt for 2	2.8 %
	Italian Spinach & Ricotta Cannelloni	2.8 %
	Italian Tomato & Mozzarella Pasta Bake	2.8 %
	Kids Cheese Ravioli	2.8 %
	Smartprice Lasagne	2.8 %
	Smartprice Minced Beef & Onion Pies	2.8 %
	Taste of America Loaded Hot Dog Style Chilli Bake	2.8 %
	Taste of America Mouth-Watering Beefy Burritos	2.8 %
	Tomato & Mozzarella Pasta Bake for 4	2.8 %
	Beef Lasagne for 4	2.9 %
	Chicken & Mushrooms	2.9 %
	Classic Moussaka	2.9 %
	Extra Special West Country Beef Lasagne for 2	2.9 %
	Fresh Tastes Kitchen Chicken Tikka Masala & Rice	2.9 %
	Fresh Tastes Kitchen Malaysian Chicken Curry	2.9 %
	Fresh Tastes Kitchen Red Thai King Prawn Curry & Noodles	2.9 %
	Good & Balanced Italian Chicken & Tomato Wholemeal Pasta	2.9 %
	Good & Counted Beef Lasagne	2.9 %
	Kids Cheese & Creamy Tomato Pasta	2.9 %
	Kids Roast Chicken & Gravy Pie	2.9 %
	Pub Classics Chicken Jalfrezi with Lemon Rice	2.9 %
	Sizzler Fajita Chicken for 2	2.9 %

Ready Meals - by brand (continued)

Brand	Label	% Sugar
ASDA	Smartprice Bolognese Pasta Bake	2.9 %
	Vegetable Chow Mein	2.9 %
	Classic All Day Breakfast	3.0 %
	Extra Special Venison Casserole with Sloe Gin & Potato	3.0 %
	Fresh Tastes Kitchen Piri Piri Chicken & Rice	3.0 %
	Fresh Tastes Kitchen Red Thai Chicken Curry & Rice	3.0 %
	Fresh Tastes Kitchen Sweet Chilli Beef Noodles	3.0 %
	Good & Balanced Moroccan Lamb Meatballs with Cous Cous	3.0 %
	Good & Balanced Tandoori Chicken with Basmati Rice	3.0 %
	Good & Counted Ham Hock with Root Mash	3.0 %
	Good & Counted Spinach & Ricotta Cannelloni	3.0 %
	Italian Sausage Pasta Bake	3.0 %
	Italian Sausage Pasta Bake for 2	3.0 %
	Sausage Pasta Bake for 4	3.0 %
	Vegetarian Pepper & Courgette Lasagne	3.0 %
	Vegetarian Sweet Potato & Mozzarella Bakes	3.0 %
Aunt Bessie's	Cheese & Onion Potato Bake	0.7 %
	Vegetarian Toad in the Hole	1.2 %
	Deep Filled Chicken Pie	1.8 %
	Large Toad in the Hole	1.8 %
	Deep Filled Steak Pie	2.0 %
	Toad in the Hole	2.0 %
	Mini Toad in the Hole	2.3 %

Ready Meals - by brand (continued)

Brand	Label	% Sugar
Baxters	Malaysian Inspired Chicken Laksa	3.0 %
Birds Eye	Homebake Cheese & Onion Rolls	0.6 %
	Puff Pastry British Steak Pies	1.1 %
	Puff Pastry Chicken & Ham Pies	1.1 %
	Four Cheese Penne Pasta	1.4 %
	Prawn Curry with Rice	1.5 %
	Shortcrust Meat & Potato Pies	1.5 %
	Shortcrust Steak Pies	1.5 %
	Stir Your Senses South Indian Chicken Curry	1.5 %
	Stir Your Senses Tagliatelle con Porcini	1.5 %
	Stir Your Senses Thai Chicken with Basmati Rice	1.5 %
	Traditional Beef Dinner	1.5 %
	Creamy Cheese Penne Pasta	1.8 %
	Shortcrust Chicken Pies	1.8 %
	Steamfresh Creamy Cheese Penne Pasta	1.8 %
	Stir Your Senses Rigatoni alla Carbonara	1.8 %
	Stir Your Senses Pappardelle alla Bolognese	1.9 %
	Macaroni with Cheese & Ham	2.0 %
	Shortcrust Creamy Chicken Pies	2.0 %
	Chicken Curry with Rice	2.2 %
	Chicken Jalfrezi with Rice	2.2 %
	Chicken Tikka Masala with Rice	2.2 %
	Stir Your Senses Gnocchi con Gorgonzola e Spinaci	2.4 %
	Stir Your Senses Spanish Paella with Chicken and Prawn	2.5 %
	Stir Your Senses Penne all Arrabbiata con Pollo	2.8 %

Ready Meals - by brand (continued)

Brand	Label	% Sugar
Birds Eye	Mediterranean Vegetable Penne Pasta	3.0 %
	Steamfresh Mediterranean Vegetable Pasta	3.0 %
	Traditional Beef with Homestyle Gravy	3.0 %
Bisto	Cottage Pie	0.6 %
	Shepherd's Pie	0.8 %
	Bangers & Mash	1.0 %
	Chicken Hotpot	1.1 %
	Minced Beef Hotpot	1.2 %
	Roast Lamb Dinner	1.4 %
	Roast Beef Dinner	1.5 %
	Roast Chicken Dinner	1.5 %
	Beef Lasagne	1.9 %
	Roast Turkey Dinner	1.9 %
	Toad In The Hole	2.1 %
Cauldron	South American Empanadas	1.9 %
Charlie Bingham's	Chicken Kiev	0.4 %
	Breton Chicken	0.7 %
	Chicken Wrapped in Prosciutto	0.7 %
	Beef Stroganoff & Rice	0.8 %
	Chicken en Croute	0.8 %
	Steak & Ale Pies	0.8 %
	Chicken Breasts with White Wine Sauce & Mash	0.9 %
	Beef Bourguignon & Potato Dauphinoise	1.0 %
	Chicken & Mushroom Pies	1.0 %
	Chicken & Mushroom Risotto	1.3 %

Ready Meals - by brand (continued)

Brand	Label	% Sugar
Charlie Bingham's	Spaghetti Bolognese	1.3 %
	Chilli con Carne & Mexican Rice	1.4 %
	Cottage Pie	1.4 %
	Fish Pie	1.5 %
	Chicken Jalfrezi & Pilau Rice	1.7 %
	Shepherd's Pie	1.9 %
	Spaghetti Carbonara	1.9 %
	Macaroni Cheese	2.0 %
	Spanish Chicken & Roasted Potatoes	2.0 %
	Thai Green Chicken Curry	2.0 %
	Chicken Korma & Pilau Rice	2.2 %
	Lasagne	2.2 %
	Moussaka	2.2 %
	Thai Red Chicken Curry & Fragrant Rice	2.2 %
	Salmon en Croute	2.3 %
	Spinach & Ricotta Cannelloni	2.4 %
	Chicken Tikka Masala & Pilau Rice	2.5 %
	Paella with Chicken, King Prawns & Chorizo	2.5 %
Cook	Salmon & Dill Tart	0.5 %
	Pork Dijon	0.6 %
	Tarka Dal	0.8 %
	Chicken Catalan	0.9 %
	Chicken Pho	0.9 %
	Classic Fish Pie	0.9 %
	Risotto with Porcini Mushrooms, Lemon and Sage Butter	1.1 %

Ready Meals - by brand (continued)

Brand	Label	% Sugar
Cook	Rosemary Chicken with Portobello Mushroom & Pearl Barley Risotto	1.2 %
	Lemon Chicken Risotto Family Meal	1.3 %
	Salmon and Asparagus Gratin	1.3 %
	Salmon Wellington	1.3 %
	Liver, Bacon and Onions	1.5 %
	Chicken Alexander	1.7 %
	Coq au Vin	1.7 %
	Sea Bass with Asparagus & Linguine in Lobster & Saffron Bisque	1.7 %
	Slow-cooked Rump Beef with Brandy	1.8 %
	Thai Style Chicken Patties	1.8 %
	Beef Stroganoff	1.9 %
	Chicken & Pancetta Pie	1.9 %
	Chicken, Ham and Leek Pie	2.0 %
	Kids Cottage Pie	2.0 %
	Lamb Casserole with New Potatoes	2.0 %
	Spaghetti Bolognese	2.0 %
	Steak and Red Wine Pie	2.0 %
	Kids Chicken and Mash Pie	2.1 %
	Nasi Goreng For 2	2.1 %
	Pot Roast Chicken	2.1 %
	Steak, Mushroom & Merlot Pie	2.1 %
	Chicken Dijon	2.2 %
	Saag Paneer	2.2 %
	Yellow Malaysian Fish Curry	2.2 %

Ready Meals - by brand (continued)

Brand	Label	% Sugar
Cook	Chicken Korma	2.3 %
	Kids Fish Pie	2.4 %
	Lamb Moussaka	2.4 %
	Nasi Goreng	2.4 %
	Thai Butternut Squash Soup	2.4 %
	Linguine Carbonara Family Meal	2.5 %
	Chilli con Carne	2.6 %
	Macaroni Cheese	2.6 %
	Cottage Pie	2.7 %
	Shepherd's Pie	2.7 %
	Chicken Noodle Laksa For 2	2.8 %
	Lamb Hotpot	2.8 %
	Red Thai Chicken Curry	2.9 %
	Beef Bolognese Pasta Bake Family Meal	3.0 %
	Japanese Salmon	3.0 %
	Keralan Prawn Curry	3.0 %
Dolmio	Carbonara Pasta Vista	1.3 %
	Creamy Mushroom Pasta Vista	1.3 %
	Bolognese Pasta Vista	2.6 %
	Tomato & Basil Pasta Vista	2.9 %
DS Gluten Free	Bonta d' Italia Lasagne	2.4 %
	Quiche Lorraine	2.5 %
Easy Bean	African Palava	2.0 %
	Indian Sambar	2.2 %
	Spanish Puchero	2.6 %

Ready Meals - by brand (continued)

Brand	Label	% Sugar
Easy Bean	French Cuisinés	3.0 %
Fray Bentos	Classic Steak & Kidney Pie	0.4 %
	Deep Fill Just Steak Pie	0.4 %
	Tender Just Steak Pie	0.4 %
	Just Chicken Pies	0.5 %
	Just Steak Pudding	0.5 %
	Steak & Kidney Pudding	0.5 %
	Deep Fill Chicken & Mushroom Pie	0.6 %
	Deep Fill Steak & Ale Pie	0.9 %
	Gentle Minced Beef & Onion Pie	1.2 %
	Hunger Burster Beef Stew & Dumplings	1.9 %
	Hunger Burster Meatballs & Pasta	3.0 %
Genius	Gluten Free Chicken & Gravy Pies	1.9 %
	Gluten Free Steak Pies	2.6 %
	Gluten Free Vegetable Curry Pies	2.8 %
Georgia's Choice	Chicken & Mushroom Crispy Bake	0.6 %
	Fish Cakes	0.9 %
	Mexican Bean Bake	2.3 %
	Beef Lasagne	2.9 %
Gino's	Deep Pan Pepperoni Pizza	2.9 %
Ginsters	Steak Pie	0.8 %
	Chicken & Bacon Pasty	1.1 %
	Chicken & Mushroom Pie	1.3 %
	Steak & Kidney Pie	1.5 %
	Original Cornish Pasty	1.8 %

Ready Meals - by brand (continued)

Brand	Label	% Sugar
Giovanni Rana	Lasagne Bolognese	3.0 %
Heinz	Big Chicken Casserole with Chunky Potatoes	1.5 %
	Big Chilli Con Carne with Chunky Wedges	1.9 %
	Big Pasta Bolognese with Chunky Pasta	1.9 %
	Big Beef Hotpot with Chunky Veg	2.6 %
Higgidy	Little Mushroom, Feta & Spinach Pie	0.9 %
	Crustless Smoked English Bacon & Mature Cheddar Quiche	1.0 %
	Little Smoked Bacon and Cheddar Quiche	1.1 %
	Little Spinach & Roasted Red Pepper Quiche	1.1 %
	Spinach, Feta & Toasted Pine Nut Pie	1.5 %
	Cauliflower Cheese Pie with Chestnut Crumble	1.8 %
Holland's	Guinness Steak Pie	1.5 %
	Meat Pies	1.5 %
	Pub Classics Chicken & Ham Pie	2.1 %
	Lancashire Hotpots	2.2 %
	Steak & Kidney Puddings	2.3 %
	Potato & Meat Pies	2.4 %
	Steak & Kidney Pies	2.6 %
	Minced Beef & Onion Pies	2.7 %
	Pub Classics Peppered Steak Pie	2.9 %
Hunger Breaks	The Full Monty	2.6 %
Hungry Joe's	Blazin' Beef Chilli & Spicy Rice	1.7 %
	Chicken Curry with Rice & Naan	2.3 %

Ready Meals – by brand (continued)

Brand	Label	% Sugar
Hungry Joe's	Joe Vs. Vindaloo with Rice & Naan	2.3 %
	Cajun Chicken & Spicy Rice	2.8 %
	Mighty Meatball Pasta Feast	2.8 %
John West	Steam Pot Tuna with Chilli & Garlic and Spicy Red Pepper Couscous	0.8 %
	Steam Pot Tuna with Basil and Sun-Dried Tomato Couscous	1.2 %
	Steam Pot Tuna with Lemon & Thyme and Tomato & Black Olive Couscous	1.2 %
	Steam Pot Tuna with Mixed Peppercorn and Tomato & Black Olive Couscous	1.4 %
	Steam Pot Tuna with Coriander & Cumin and Thyme & Coriander Couscous	1.5 %
	Light Lunch Italian Style Tuna Salad	1.8 %
	Steam Pot Tuna with Soy & Ginger and Mushroom Couscous	2.0 %
	Light Lunch French Style Tuna Salad	2.3 %
	Light Lunch Mexican Style Tuna Salad	2.7 %
Kingston Town	Jerk Chicken with Rice & Peas	0.5 %
	Curry Mutton with Rice & Gungo Peas	1.1 %
Kirsty's	Thai Chilli Chicken with Rice Noodles	0.4 %
	Beef Lasagne with Rich Bolognese Sauce	1.1 %
	Sausage And Sweet Potato Mash	1.4 %
	Chicken Tikka Masala with Brown Basmati Rice	2.2 %
	Spanish Chicken with Brown Rice	2.3 %
	Moroccan Vegetables with Quinoa	2.5 %
Levi Roots	Jamaican Coconut Chicken Curry with Rice & Peas	2.1 %

Ready Meals - by brand (continued)

Brand	Label	% Sugar
Levi Roots	Caribbean Curried Chicken Noodles	2.4 %
	Caribbean Hot Chilli Beef with Seasoned Rice	2.7 %
Linda McCartney	Cannelloni	1.1 %
	Farmhouse Pies	1.4 %
	Mushroom and Ale Pie	2.0 %
	Asparagus & Leek Tartlets	2.2 %
	Butternut Squash & Goats Cheese Tartlet	2.2 %
	Cheese & Leek Plaits	2.2 %
	Cheese, Leek & Red Onion Plaits	2.6 %
	Lentil & Vegetable Cottage Pie	2.7 %
	Vegetarian Sausage & Vegetable Hot Pot	2.8 %
Little Dish	Fish Pie with Salmon and Pollock	0.9 %
	Fisherman's Pie with Salmon and Pollock	1.8 %
	Chicken and Butternut Squash Pie	1.9 %
	Chunky Chicken Pot Roast	1.9 %
	Mild Beef Chilli & Rice	1.9 %
	Mediterranean Cod and Tomato Casserole	2.1 %
	Pasta Seashells with Salmon and Broccoli	2.3 %
	Mini Cheese Ravioli in Tomato & Veg Sauce	2.4 %
	Spaghetti with Mini Meatballs	2.4 %
	Mild Chicken Curry with Rice	2.7 %
	Pork and Apple Bites with Beans	2.7 %
	British Lamb Hotpot	2.8 %
	Classic Beef Lasagne	2.8 %
	Cottage Pie with Seven Veg	2.8 %

Ready Meals - by brand (continued)

Brand	Label	% Sugar
Little Dish	Alphabet Pasta Bolognese	3.0 %
Look What We Found!	Staffordshire Chicken Casserole	0.2 %
	Tees Valley Beef in Black Velvet Ale	1.3 %
	Tees Valley Beef Casserole	1.4 %
	Chilli Con Carne & Long Grain Rice	1.7 %
	Staffordshire Chicken Korma	2.0 %
	Staffordshire Chicken Thai Green Curry	2.5 %
	Staffordshire Chicken Thai Red Curry	2.8 %
	Yorkshire Pork Sausage Casserole	2.8 %
Low Low	Beef Hotpot	1.3 %
	Chicken in White Wine Sauce with Pasta	2.1 %
	Chicken Biryani	2.4 %
	Chicken & Chorizo Paella	2.9 %
	Chicken Tomato & Basil Pasta	3.0 %
Morrisons	M Kitchen Chinese Takeaway Egg Fried Rice	0.0 %
	M Kitchen Tastes of Home Liver & Bacon with Mash	0.1 %
	Steak & Ale Puff Pastry Pie	0.1 %
	Savers Chicken in White Sauce	0.2 %
	M Kitchen Tastes of Home Sausage & Mash	0.3 %
	Signature Coq Au Vin	0.3 %
	Savers Cottage Pie	0.4 %
	Steak Puff Pastry Pie	0.4 %
	M Kitchen Italian Chicken Risotto	0.5 %
	M Kitchen Tastes of Home Braised Beef & Mash	0.5 %

Ready Meals - by brand (continued)

Brand	Label	% Sugar
Morrisons	M Kitchen Tastes of Home Slow-Cooked Beef Brisket with Gravy	0.5 %
	M Kitchen Tex Mex Southern Fried-Style Chicken with Curly Fries	0.5 %
	Steak & Ale Large Puff Pastry Pie	0.5 %
	Steak Large Shortcrust Pie	0.5 %
	M Kitchen Tastes of Home Chicken & Mushroom Cumberland Pie	0.6 %
	M Kitchen Tastes of Home Fisherman's Pie	0.6 %
	Steak Small Puff Pastry Pie	0.6 %
	Classic Fish & Chips	0.7 %
	M Kitchen Fresh Ideas Mini Roast Chicken Dinner	0.7 %
	M Kitchen Fresh Ideas Smoky Bacon Chicken	0.7 %
	M Kitchen Italian Macaroni Cheese with Bacon	0.7 %
	M Kitchen Tastes of Home Slow-Cooked Beef Rib in Gravy	0.7 %
	Signature British Steak Diane	0.7 %
	Signature Smoked Haddock & King Prawn Fish Pie	0.7 %
	Steak & Kidney Small Shortcrust Pie	0.7 %
	M Kitchen Italian Ham & Mushroom Tagliatelle	0.8 %
	NuMe Chicken Dinner	0.8 %
	Cumberland Pie	0.9 %
	M Kitchen Tastes of Home Braised Steak & Mash	0.9 %
	Signature British Rump Steak Stroganoff & Buttered Rice	0.9 %
	Signature Cottage Pie with Real Ale Gravy	0.9 %
	Signature King Prawn & Slow Roasted Tomato Linguine	0.9 %

Ready Meals - by brand (continued)

Brand	Label	% Sugar
Morrisons	Chicken & Mushroom Puff Pastry Pie	1.0 %
	Classic Steak Pie & Chips	1.0 %
	M Kitchen Tastes of Home Beef Casserole	1.0 %
	M Kitchen Tastes of Home Cottage Pie	1.0 %
	Signature Wiltshire-Cured Ham & Chestnut Mushroom Tagliatelle	1.0 %
	Chicken & Bacon Carbonara	1.1 %
	Chicken, Ham & Leek Puff Pastry Pie	1.1 %
	Dumpling Topped Minced Steak Puff Pastry Pie	1.1 %
	M Kitchen Italian Macaroni Cheese	1.1 %
	M Kitchen Italian Spaghetti Carbonara	1.1 %
	M Kitchen Tastes of Home Cumberland Pie	1.1 %
	M Kitchen Tastes of Home Minced Beef Hotpot	1.1 %
	M Kitchen Tastes of Home Chicken with Leeks, Bacon & Roast Potatoes	1.2 %
	Minced Beef & Onion Puff Pastry Pie	1.2 %
	Signature Maris Piper Dauphinoise Potatoes	1.2 %
	Steak Shortcrust Pie	1.2 %
	Cheese & Onion Small Quiche	1.3 %
	Homestyle Lamb Dinner	1.3 %
	Just For Kids Bangers & Mash	1.3 %
	NuMe Beef in Ale with Mash	1.3 %
	NuMe Cumberland Pie	1.3 %
	Savers Irish Stew	1.3 %
	M Kitchen Fresh Ideas Honey & Mustard Chicken	1.4 %
	M Kitchen Fresh Ideas Tandoori Chicken	1.4 %
	M Kitchen Italian Beef Lasagne	1.4 %

Ready Meals - by brand (continued)

Brand	Label	% Sugar
Morrisons	M Kitchen Italian Bolognese Pasta Bake	1.4 %
	M Kitchen Oriental Special Chicken Fried Rice	1.4 %
	M Kitchen Tastes of Home Chicken Dinner with Stuffing	1.4 %
	M Kitchen Tastes of Home Corned Beef Hatch	1.4 %
	Minced Steak & Onion Shortcrust Pie	1.4 %
	Signature Maple-Cured Bacon & Gruyere Tart	1.4 %
	Signature Wild Mushroom & West Country Cheddar Tart	1.4 %
	M Kitchen Italian Bolognese Pasta Melt	1.5 %
	M Kitchen Italian Spaghetti Bolognese	1.5 %
	M Kitchen Tastes of Home Roast Chicken Dinner	1.5 %
	M Kitchen Tastes of Home Shepherd's Pie	1.5 %
	Macaroni Cheese	1.5 %
	Quiche Lorraine	1.5 %
	Savers Macaroni Cheese	1.5 %
	Cheese & Broccoli Quiche	1.6 %
	Homestyle Chicken Dinner	1.6 %
	Just For Kids Chicken Dinner	1.6 %
	M Kitchen Chicken Tikka Biryani	1.6 %
	M Kitchen Fresh Ideas Piri Piri Chicken	1.6 %
	M Kitchen Italian Lasagne	1.6 %
	M Kitchen Tastes of Home Roast Beef Dinner	1.6 %
	Quiche Lorraine Small	1.6 %
	Savers Cheese & Onion Quiche	1.6 %
	Tomato & Cheese Crustless Quiche	1.6 %
	Classic Sausage & Chips	1.7 %

Ready Meals - by brand (continued)

Brand	Label	% Sugar
Morrisons	M Kitchen Tastes of Home Potato Gratin	1.7 %
	M Kitchen Tex Mex Family Chilli Con Carne & Rice	1.7 %
	Savers Cheese & Bacon Quiche	1.7 %
	Steak & Kidney Shortcrust Pie	1.7 %
	Cheese & Onion Crustless Quiche	1.8 %
	Just for Kids Cottage Pie	1.8 %
	M Kitchen Fresh Ideas Mexican Chicken	1.8 %
	M Kitchen Indian Chicken Pasanda & Pilau Rice	1.8 %
	M Kitchen Italian Chicken & Bacon Pasta Bake	1.8 %
	M Kitchen Tastes of Home Minced Lamb Casserole	1.8 %
	M Kitchen Vegetarian Vegetable Pasta Bake	1.8 %
	Signature Cauliflower Cheese with Davidstow Cheddar	1.8 %
	Bacon & Leek Small Quiche	1.9 %
	Classic Steak let & Chips	1.9 %
	M Kitchen Indian Chicken Madras & Pilau Rice	1.9 %
	M Kitchen Tex Mex Chilli Beef Burrito	1.9 %
	NuMe Chicken Tikka Masala & Pilau Rice	1.9 %
	Homestyle Liver & Onions	2.0 %
	M Kitchen Oriental Green Thai Chicken Curry with Jasmine Rice	2.0 %
	M Kitchen Tastes of Home Slow-Cooked Lamb Shank with Mint Gravy	2.0 %
	Signature Brie & Pancetta Tart	2.0 %
	Signature British Lamb Moussaka	2.0 %
	Spinach & Ricotta Quiche	2.0 %

Ready Meals – by brand (continued)

Brand	Label	% Sugar
Morrisons	Homestyle Beef Dinner	2.1 %
	Just For Kids Chicken Casserole	2.1 %
	M Kitchen Oriental Chicken Chow Mein	2.1 %
	NuMe Cheese & Onion Quiche	2.1 %
	Quiche Lorraine Crustless	2.1 %
	Signature Shepherd's Pie with Leeks	2.1 %
	Tomato, Bacon & Mushroom Quiche	2.1 %
	Bacon & Leek Quiche	2.2 %
	M Kitchen Fresh Ideas Chicken & Chorizo Paella	2.2 %
	M Kitchen Fresh Ideas Thai Green Chicken Curry	2.2 %
	The All Day Big Breakfast	2.2 %
	M Kitchen Fresh Ideas Chicken Dinner	2.3 %
	M Kitchen Indian Chicken Bhuna & Pilau Rice	2.3 %
	M Kitchen Italian Meat Feast Pasta Melt	2.3 %
	M Kitchen Tastes of Home Minced Lamb Hotpot	2.3 %
	M Kitchen Tex Mex Chilli Con Carne & Rice	2.3 %
	M Kitchen Tex Mex Smokin' Mexican-Style Chicken	2.3 %
	NuMe Red Thai Chicken Curry & Rice	2.3 %
	M Kitchen Fresh Ideas King Prawn Linguini	2.4 %
	M Kitchen Italian Penne Bolognese Bake	2.4 %
	M Kitchen Tastes of Home Minced Beef & Potatoes	2.4 %
	Cheese & Onion Quiche	2.5 %
	Just For Kids Fish Pie	2.5 %
	Just for Kids Spaghetti Bolognese	2.5 %
	M Kitchen Italian Chicken Lasagne	2.5 %

Ready Meals – by brand (continued)

Brand	Label	% Sugar
Morrisons	M Kitchen Tastes of Home Slow-Cooked Lamb Shank in a Red Wine & Rosemary Gravy	2.5 %
	M Kitchen Tex Mex Spicy Chicken Enchilada	2.5 %
	Mexican Chicken	2.5 %
	NuMe Chilli con Carne with Rice	2.5 %
	Signature Beef Bourguignon	2.5 %
	M Kitchen Indian Chicken Rogan Josh & Pilau Rice	2.6 %
	M Kitchen Indian Tandoori Chicken & Pilau Rice	2.6 %
	M Kitchen Italian Chicken & Ham Pasta Bake	2.6 %
	M Kitchen Italian Three Cheese Pasta Melt	2.6 %
	M Kitchen Oriental Chinese Chicken Curry & Egg Fried Rice	2.6 %
	Savers Spaghetti Bolognese	2.6 %
	M Kitchen Indian Chicken Jalfrezi & Pilau Rice	2.7 %
	M Kitchen Indian Takeaway Aloo Gobi Saag	2.7 %
	M Kitchen Indian Takeaway Korma & Tikka Masala Meal for 2	2.7 %
	M Kitchen Tex Mex Blazin' Chicken Burrito	2.7 %
	M Kitchen Italian King Prawn Linguine	2.8 %
	M Kitchen Italian Lasagne	2.8 %
	M Kitchen Italian Vegetable Lasagne	2.8 %
	NuMe Lasagne	2.8 %
	Savers Beef Lasagne	2.8 %
	Signature Aberdeen Angus Lasagne	2.8 %
	M Kitchen Fresh Ideas Beef in Ale	2.9 %
	M Kitchen Fresh Ideas Moroccan Chicken	2.9 %
	M Kitchen Tex Mex Sizzlin' Salsa Chicken	2.9 %

Ready Meals – by brand (continued)

Brand	Label	% Sugar
Morrisons	M Kitchen Vegetarian Paneer Jalfrezi with Pilau Rice	2.9 %
	NuMe Quiche Lorraine	2.9 %
	M Kitchen Fresh Ideas Chicken en Croute	3.0 %
	M Kitchen Indian Chicken Tikka Masala & Pilau Rice	3.0 %
Mr. Brains	Pork Faggots	1.3 %
Mumtaz	Chicken Dopiaza & Pilau Rice	0.1 %
	Chicken Karahi & Pilau Rice	0.2 %
	Chicken Korma & Pilau Rice	0.3 %
	Chicken Tikka Masala & Pilau Rice	0.5 %
	Daal Karahi & Pilau Rice	1.1 %
	Keema Mattar Karahi & Pilau Rice	1.5 %
Our Little Secret	Delightful Carrot & Herb Rice	0.7 %
	Exotic Seafood Paella	1.1 %
	Flavoursome Curried Chicken Rice	3.0 %
Peter's	Steak & Kidney Pie	0.4 %
	Premier Steak Pie	0.7 %
	Premier Steak & Kidney Pie	1.1 %
	Premier Roast Chicken Pie	1.2 %
Pieminister	Moo Pie	0.1 %
	The Free Ranger Pie	0.2 %
	Matador Pie	1.4 %
	Chicken of Aragon Pie	1.6 %
	The Deerstalker Pie	1.8 %
	Fungi Chicken Pie	1.9 %
	Cheeky Chick Pie Pot	2.0 %

Ready Meals - by brand (continued)

Brand	Label	% Sugar
Pieminister	Wild Shroom Pie	2.1 %
	Shamrock Pie	2.3 %
	Kate & Sidney Pie	2.6 %
	Matador Pie Pot	2.6 %
	Moo & Blue Pie	2.6 %
	Moo & Brew Pie Pot	2.7 %
Pooles	Potato & Meat Pies	1.8 %
	Cheese & Onion Pies	2.1 %
	Minced Beef & Onion Pies	2.7 %
Princes	Italian Tuna Salad	0.4 %
	Chicken Casserole	0.8 %
	Chicken in White Sauce	0.8 %
	Creamy Cheese Tuna Pasta Bake	1.5 %
	Hot Chicken Curry	1.7 %
	Mild Chicken Curry	2.0 %
	Chilli Con Carne	2.6 %
	Mexican Tuna Salad	2.8 %
Pukka-Pies	Steak & Ale Pie	0.8 %
	Large Potato and Meat Pie	0.9 %
	Large Steak & Kidney Pie	1.0 %
	Family All Steak Pie	1.1 %
	Peppered Steak Pie	1.1 %
	Steak & Cheese Pie	1.1 %
	Family Chicken & Gravy Pies	1.2 %
	Family Steak & Onion Pie	1.3 %
	Large Beef and Onion Pie	1.3 %

Ready Meals - by brand (continued)

Brand	Label	% Sugar
Pukka-Pies	Large All Steak Pie	1.5 %
	Frozen Family Chicken & Veg Pies	1.6 %
	Frozen Family Steak Pies	1.6 %
	Minced Steak & Onion Pies	1.6 %
	Large Chicken Balti Pie	1.7 %
	Large Potato, Cheese & Onion Pie	1.7 %
	Microwaveable All Steak Pie	1.7 %
	Steak & Kidney Pudding	1.7 %
	Chicken & Vegetable Pies	1.8 %
	Beef and Onion Pukka Pasty	2.0 %
	Large Stand-Up Pasty	2.2 %
	Microwaveable Chicken Pie	2.3 %
	Potato, Cheese & Onion Pasty	2.3 %
	Large Chicken & Mushroom Pie	2.7 %
Quorn	Meat Free Spaghetti Bolognese	0.9 %
	Meat Free Chicken Style & Mushroom Pie	1.4 %
	Meat Free Cottage Pie	1.4 %
	Meat Free Curry & Rice	1.6 %
	Meat Free Low Fat Sausages	1.7 %
	Meat Free Italian Pasta Bake	1.8 %
	Meat Free Chef's Selection Steak & Gravy Pudding	2.0 %
	Meat Free Steak Style Slice	2.0 %
	Meat Free Stew & Dumplings	2.0 %
	Meat Free Tikka Masala With Rice	2.2 %
	Meat Free Steak Style Pie	2.3 %
	Meat Free Pasty	2.4 %

Ready Meals - by brand (continued)

Brand	Label	% Sugar
Quorn	Meat Free Lasagne	2.5 %
	Meat Free Mexican Chilli Burrito	2.6 %
	Meat Free Piri Piri & Rice	2.9 %
	Meat Free Chicken Style & Leek Pie	3.0 %
	Meat Free Chilli & Wedges	3.0 %
Sainsbury's	Basics Cottage Pie	0.5 %
	Chicken & Mushroom Casserole	0.5 %
	Chicken in White Sauce	0.5 %
	Classic Chicken Supreme	0.5 %
	Chicken & Mushroom Risotto	0.6 %
	Pub Specials Chicken, Ham Hock & Leek Pies	0.8 %
	Steak Family Pie	0.9 %
	Chicken & Gravy Family Pie	1.0 %
	Classic Shepherd's Pie	1.1 %
	Pub Specials Chicken in Red Wine & Thyme Sauce	1.1 %
	Chicken Jalfrezi	1.2 %
	Chicken Korma	1.3 %
	Pub Specials Chicken & Bacon Risotto	1.3 %
	Pub Specials Steak & Ale Pies	1.3 %
	Basics Beef Curry with Rice	1.4 %
	Classic Chicken Dinner	1.4 %
	Basics Beef In Gravy	1.5 %
	Basics Macaroni Cheese	1.5 %
	Classic Chicken Hotpot Dinner	1.5 %
	Pub Specials Gammon Hock in a Cider Sauce with Mustard Mash	1.5 %

Ready Meals - by brand (continued)

Brand	Label	% Sugar
Sainsbury's	Chickpea Dahl	1.6 %
	Classic Gammon & Parsley Sauce	1.6 %
	Pub Specials Creamy Peppercorn Chicken	1.6 %
	Chicken Balti	1.7 %
	Be Good Chicken Curry with Rice	1.8 %
	Be Good Lemon Chicken Risotto	1.8 %
	Chicken & Mushroom Pies	1.8 %
	Steak & Kidney Pies	1.8 %
	Basics Chicken & Vegetable Pies	1.9 %
	Basics Chicken Curry with Rice	1.9 %
	Basics Minced Beef Hotpot	1.9 %
	Classic Beef Dinner	2.0 %
	Basics Chilli con Carne with Rice	2.1 %
	Be Good Beef Lasagne	2.1 %
	Classic Lamb Dinner	2.2 %
	Pub Specials Beef Lasagne	2.2 %
	Pub Specials Slow Cooked Beef in Red Wine with Gratin Potatoes	2.2 %
	Basics Chilli con Carne	2.3 %
	Basics Toad in the Hole	2.3 %
	Beef Stew & Dumplings Dinner	2.3 %
	Classic Liver & Bacon Dinner	2.3 %
	Basics Prawn Curry with Rice	2.4 %
	Chicken Jalfrezi with Pilau Rice	2.4 %
	Chicken Korma with Rice	2.7 %
	Chip Shop Chicken Curry	2.7 %

Ready Meals - by brand (continued)

Brand	Label	% Sugar
Sainsbury's	Italian Beef Lasagne	2.7 %
	Butter Chicken with Rice	2.8 %
	Vegetarian Vegetable Lasagne	2.8 %
	Chickpea & Chorizo Stew	2.9 %
	Vegetable Pies	2.9 %
	Basics Spaghetti Bolognese	3.0 %
	Beef Bolognese	3.0 %
Sharwood's	Chinese Chicken Rice	0.8 %
	Chicken Curry with Rice	1.0 %
	Chinese Chicken Curry with Rice	1.5 %
	Lamb Biryani	1.7 %
	Chicken Korma with Rice	2.0 %
	Chicken Chow Mein	2.1 %
	Chicken Tikka Masala with Rice	3.0 %
Smart-GF Kids	Brilliant Bolognese	0.8 %
	Kooky Korma	1.6 %
Stagg	Homestead Minced Chili with Beans	2.2 %
	Classic Chili con Carne	3.0 %
	Dynamite Hot Chili con Carne	3.0 %
	Silverado Beef Chili con Carne	3.0 %
Tasty Favourites	Chicken & Mushrooms With Rice	0.5 %
	Chinese Chicken Curry & Rice	1.2 %
	Beef Hot Pot	1.5 %
	Chilli Con Carne	1.6 %
	Chicken Korma	1.9 %

Ready Meals - by brand (continued)

Brand	Label	% Sugar
Tasty Favourites	Bolognese Pasta	2.1 %
	Chicken Tikka	2.6 %
Tesco	Everyday Value Chicken in White Sauce	0.1 %
	Finest Crab, Rocket & Chilli Linguine	0.1 %
	Al Fresco Chicken & Chorizo Paella	0.3 %
	Finest King Prawn Spaghetti	0.3 %
	Finest Smoked Haddock Risotto	0.3 %
	Takeaway No 26 Vegetable Chow Mein	0.3 %
	Everyday Value Chilled Cottage Pie	0.4 %
	Chicken Curry	0.5 %
	Everyday Value Sausage And Mash	0.5 %
	Tex Mex Chicken Fajitas	0.5 %
	Chicken in White Sauce	0.6 %
	Everyday Value Fisherman's Pie	0.6 %
	British Classics Fish Pie	0.7 %
	Finest Chicken Madeira and Braised Rice with Mushrooms	0.7 %
	Finest Spaghetti Carbonara	0.7 %
	Al Fresco Polenta & Smoked Mozzarella	0.8 %
	Chicken Fajita Puff Pastry Pie	0.8 %
	Everyday Value Cheese Omelettes	0.8 %
	Finest Aberdeen Angus Cottage Pie	0.8 %
	Finest Beef Stroganoff with Wild Rice	0.8 %
	Finest Slow Cooked Steak Ragu with Pappardelle	0.8 %
	Healthy Living Chicken Chow Mein	0.8 %
	Italian Creamy Cheese & Bacon Spaghetti	0.8 %

Ready Meals - by brand (continued)

Brand	Label	% Sugar
Tesco	Takeaway Chinese Chicken Curry with Egg Fried Rice & Prawn Crackers	0.8 %
	British Classics Beef Roast Dinner	0.8 %
	British Classics Minced Lamb Hotpot	0.8 %
	Classic Italian Tuna Pasta Bake	0.9 %
	Everyday Value Cheese & Onion Quiche	0.9 %
	Family Favourites Mild Chilli con Carne with Rice	0.9 %
	Finest Cod & Crab Bake	0.9 %
	Finest Slow Cooked West Country Large Steak Pie	0.9 %
	British Classics Beef Casserole & Dumplings	0.9 %
	Classic Italian Macaroni Cheese	1.0 %
	Creamy Chicken & Bacon Puff Pastry Pie	1.0 %
	Finest Chicken with Italian Pancetta & Mozzarella	1.0 %
	Finest Roast Chicken & Gravy Pie	1.0 %
	Finest Shepherds Pie	1.0 %
	Slow Cooked Steak & Kidney Suet Pudding	1.0 %
	British Classics Large Cottage Pie	1.0 %
	British Classics Minced Beef & Mash	1.0 %
	British Classics Shepherd's Pie	1.0 %
	Egg Fried Rice	1.0 %
	Takeaway No 24 Egg Fried Rice	1.0 %
	Al Fresco Chicken & Roasted Mushrooms	1.1 %
	Chicken & Mushroom Pie	1.1 %
	Everyday Value Chicken Curry	1.1 %
	Everyday Value Macaroni Cheese	1.1 %
	Family Favourites Cottage Pie	1.1 %

Ready Meals - by brand (continued)

Brand	Label	% Sugar
Tesco	Family Favourites Creamy Chicken & Bacon Casserole	1.1 %
	Finest Chicken & Beech Smoked Bacon Pasta Bake	1.1 %
	Finest Chicken & Smoked Bacon Pasta Bake	1.1 %
	Finest Slow Cooked West Country Steak Pie	1.1 %
	Finest West Country Steak Top Crust Pie	1.1 %
	Healthy Living Chicken & Bacon Pasta	1.1 %
	Healthy Living Spaghetti Bolognese	1.1 %
	Slow Cooked Steak & Kidney Shortcrust Pastry Pie	1.1 %
	Slow Cooked Steak Shortcrust Pastry Pie	1.1 %
	Thai Chicken Green Curry with Jasmine Rice	1.1 %
	British Classics Chicken Roast Dinner	1.1 %
	British Classics Sausages & Mash	1.1 %
	Special Fried Rice	1.1 %
	Chicken & Mushroom Puff Pastry Pie	1.2 %
	Everyday Value Creamy Mushroom Chicken And Rice	1.2 %
	Everyday Value Frozen Cottage Pie	1.2 %
	Everyday Value Minced Beef & Onion Pie	1.2 %
	Everyday Value Shepherds Pie	1.2 %
	Family Favourites Carbonara Pasta	1.2 %
	Modern Italian Chicken Breasts with Creamy Mushroom Sauce	1.2 %
	Slow Cooked Steak & Ale Puff Pastry Pie	1.2 %
	Slow Cooked Steak Puff Pastry Pie	1.2 %
	British Classics Chicken in Mushroom Sauce with Rice	1.2 %

Ready Meals - by brand (continued)

Brand	Label	% Sugar
Tesco	Classic Cumberland Pie	1.3 %
	Creamy Chicken & Broccoli Large Puff Pastry Pie	1.3 %
	Creamy Chicken & White Wine Shortcrust Pie	1.3 %
	Finest Vintage Cheddar Macaroni Cheese	1.3 %
	Healthy Living Salmon & Broccoli Pie	1.3 %
	Indian Butter Chicken and Pilau Rice	1.3 %
	Marinated Chicken with Buttered Courgette Rice	1.3 %
	Steak & Kidney Pie	1.3 %
	British Classics Chicken Casserole & Dumplings	1.3 %
	British Classics Cottage Pie	1.3 %
	British Classics Large Fish Pie	1.3 %
	British Classics Turkey Roast Dinner	1.3 %
	Oriental Chicken Chow Mein	1.4 %
	Beef Curry	1.4 %
	Big Night In Indian Tarka Dahl	1.4 %
	Chicken & Ham Puff Pastry Lattice	1.4 %
	Classic Chicken Dinner	1.4 %
	Classic Italian Chicken & Bacon Pasta Bake	1.4 %
	Classic Italian Spaghetti Carbonara	1.4 %
	Everyday Value Chicken & Gravy Pie	1.4 %
	Everyday Value Chicken Hotpot	1.4 %
	Everyday Value Minced Beef & Onion Pies	1.4 %
	Family Favourites Minced Beef with Potatoes	1.4 %
	Indian Tarka Dahl	1.4 %
	Minced Beef & Onion Pie	1.4 %
	Modern Italian Spicy Beef & Jalapeno Melt	1.4 %

Ready Meals - by brand (continued)

Brand	Label	% Sugar
Tesco	Oriental Green Thai Chicken Curry with Rice	1.4 %
	Spinach & Ricotta Puff Pastry Tart	1.4 %
	Steak Pie	1.4 %
	Classic Italian Chicken & Bacon Pasta Bake	1.5 %
	Classic Italian Ham & Mushroom Tagliatelle	1.5 %
	Classic Italian Spaghetti Bolognese	1.5 %
	Creamy Chicken & Bacon Large Puff Pastry Pie	1.5 %
	Finest Chicken Biriyani	1.5 %
	Finest Traditional Lasagne	1.5 %
	Healthy Living Chicken & Broccoli Pie	1.5 %
	British Classics Chicken in Red Wine Sauce with Rosemary Potatoes	1.5 %
	British Classics Cumberland Pie	1.5 %
	British Classics Minced Beef Hotpot	1.5 %
	Chicken & Gravy Shortcrust Pie	1.6 %
	Chicken, Bacon & Cheese Bakes	1.6 %
	Creamy Chicken Bakes	1.6 %
	Everyday Value Cheese Burger And Chips	1.6 %
	Finest Chicken in a White Wine Sauce with Leeks	1.6 %
	Healthy Living Cottage Pie	1.6 %
	Slow Cooked Minced Steak & Onion Shortcrust Pastry Pie	1.6 %
	British Classics Braised Beef & Mash	1.6 %
	British Classics Chicken & Stuffing Bake	1.6 %
	British Classics Liver, Bacon & Mash	1.6 %
	Al Fresco Pulled Pork in Cannellini Bean Sauce	1.7 %

Ready Meals - by brand (continued)

Brand	Label	% Sugar
Tesco	Big Night In Thai Green Chicken Curry & Jasmine Rice	1.7 %
	Chicken & Gravy Shortcrust Pastry Pie	1.7 %
	Chicken, Ham Hock, & Leek Puff Pastry Pies	1.7 %
	Classic Beef Dinner	1.7 %
	Creamy Chicken & White Wine Large Shortcrust Pie	1.7 %
	Everyday Value Spaghetti Bolognese	1.7 %
	Finest Lemon & Black Pepper Chicken Pasta	1.7 %
	Finest Spaghetti Bolognese	1.7 %
	Healthy Living Chicken & Prawn Paella	1.7 %
	Modern Italian Chilli Beef Lasagne	1.7 %
	Slow Cooked Steak & Onion Puff Pastry Lattice	1.7 %
	Slow Cooked Steak & Onion Puff Pastry Pie	1.7 %
	Slow Cooked Steak Shortcrust Pastry Pie	1.7 %
	Big Night In Chinese Chicken Chow Mein	1.7 %
	Takeaway No 25 Vegetable Chop Suey	1.7 %
	Chicken & Bacon Pies	1.8 %
	Classic Italian Large Beef Lasagne	1.8 %
	Everyday Value Minced Beef Hotpot	1.8 %
	Finest Lasagne Al Forno	1.8 %
	Finest Smoked Haddock Fishcakes	1.8 %
	Healthy Living Baked Potatoes with Cheese	1.8 %
	Healthy Living Chilli & Rice	1.8 %
	Modern Italian Creamy Prawn Linguine	1.8 %
	Slow Cooked Minced Steak & Onion Large Shortcrust Pastry Pie	1.8 %
	Steak & Ale Puff Pastry Pies	1.8 %

Ready Meals – by brand (continued)

Brand	Label	% Sugar
Tesco	Toad In The Hole	1.8 %
	Al Fresco Pea & Pancetta Risotto	1.9 %
	Big Night In Thai Red Chicken Curry & Rice	1.9 %
	Cheese & Bacon Crustless Quiche	1.9 %
	Chicken & Vegetable Pies	1.9 %
	Finest Chicken Dhansak with Pilau Rice	1.9 %
	Finest Potato Topped Chicken Pie	1.9 %
	Finest Roast Chicken & Italian Pancetta Bake	1.9 %
	Oriental Red Thai Chicken Curry with Rice	1.9 %
	Oriental Chicken & Mushroom With Egg Fried Rice	1.9 %
	Big Night In Indian Saag Aloo	2.0 %
	Chicken Tikka Masala	2.0 %
	Classic Italian Beef Lasagne	2.0 %
	Classic Lamb Hotpot	2.0 %
	Everyday Value Chicken Vegetable Pies	2.0 %
	Everyday Value Toad In The Hole	2.0 %
	Finest Chicken Chasseur	2.0 %
	Finest Lamb Rogan Josh with Pilau Rice	2.0 %
	Indian Saag Aloo	2.0 %
	Lamb Rogan Josh	2.0 %
	Small Quiche Lorraine	2.0 %
	Al Fresco Beef Stifado with Chunky Potatoes	2.0 %
	Bacon & Leek Quiche	2.1 %
	Big Night In Indian Chicken Biryani	2.1 %
	Chinese Chicken Curried Rice	2.1 %
	Classic Minced Beef Filled Yorkshire	2.1 %

Ready Meals - by brand (continued)

Brand	Label	% Sugar
Tesco	Everyday Value Macaroni Cheese	2.1 %
	Finest Beef Chianti with Rosemary Potatoes	2.1 %
	Finest Beef In Chianti with Potatoes	2.1 %
	Finest Chicken Tikka Masala & Jalfrezi Meal For 2	2.1 %
	Finest Large Lasagne Al Forno	2.1 %
	Finest Prawn Tikka Masala with Pilau Rice	2.1 %
	Healthy Living Chicken with Baby Potatoes & Vegetables	2.1 %
	Indian Chicken Korma and Pilau Rice	2.1 %
	Indian Chicken Tikka Masala With Pilau Rice	2.1 %
	Oriental Chicken & Blackbean With Egg Fried Rice	2.1 %
	Chicken Korma	2.2 %
	Classic Italian Family Beef Lasagne	2.2 %
	Classic Italian Spinach & Ricotta Cannelloni	2.2 %
	Everyday Value Bean And Cheese Melts	2.2 %
	Finest Chicken Korma with Pilau Rice	2.2 %
	Finest Cumberland Pork Sausages & Creamy Mash	2.2 %
	Finest Slow Cooked Beef with Buttered Roast Potatoes	2.2 %
	Finest Spanish Chicken with Chorizo	2.2 %
	Healthy Living Braised Beef & Root Veg Mash	2.2 %
	Healthy Living Cheese & Bacon Crustless Quiche	2.2 %
	Indian Beef Madras and Pilau Rice	2.2 %
	Quiche Lorraine	2.2 %
	Tex Mex Spicy Beef Burrito	2.2 %
	Al Fresco Broad Beans & Peas with Feta	2.2 %
	Indian Saag Bhaji	2.2 %

Ready Meals - by brand (continued)

Brand	Label	% Sugar
Tesco	Takeaway No 84 Satay Chicken	2.2 %
	Cheese & Onion Large Quiche	2.3 %
	Classic Italian Beef Cannelloni	2.3 %
	Everyday Value Chicken Curry with Vegetables	2.3 %
	Everyday Value Lasagne	2.3 %
	Finest Chicken Tikka Masala with Pilau Rice	2.3 %
	Finest Jalfrezi with Pilau Rice	2.3 %
	Finest Slow Braised Lancashire Hotpot	2.3 %
	Takeaway Thai Red & Green Chicken Curry Meal For 2	2.3 %
	Tex Mex Chicken Enchiladas	2.3 %
	Vegetable Curry	2.3 %
	Chilli Con Carne	2.4 %
	Classic All Day Breakfast	2.4 %
	Classic Italian Roasted Vegetable Lasagne	2.4 %
	Finest Malaysian Chicken Curry and Jasmine Rice	2.4 %
	Finest Spicy Pork Meatballs Pasta	2.4 %
	Healthy Living Sweet & Sour Chicken & Rice	2.4 %
	Honey & Mustard Chicken Pasta	2.4 %
	Indian Chicken Korma & Jalfrezi Meal For 2	2.4 %
	Big Night In Chinese Chicken Curry & Egg Fried Rice	2.4 %
	Big Night Time In Beef Blackbean & Egg Fried Rice	2.4 %
	Cheese & Bacon Quiche	2.5 %
	Cheese & Onion Small Quiche	2.5 %
	Classic Italian Spaghetti & Meatballs	2.5 %

Ready Meals - by brand (continued)

Brand	Label	% Sugar
Tesco	Finest Chicken Tikka with Jewelled Rice & Lime Relish	2.5 %
	Finest Mapye Cured Bacon & Gruyere Quiche	2.5 %
	Healthy Living Chicken Arrabbiatta	2.5 %
	Indian Chicken Korma With Pilau Rice	2.5 %
	Indian Chicken Tikka & Korma Meal For 2	2.5 %
	Indian Chicken Tikka Masala Pilau Rice and Bombay Potato	2.5 %
	Italian Beef Lasagne	2.5 %
	Modern Italian Chicken Breasts with Tomato & Basil Sauce	2.5 %
	Spanish Chicken & Chorizo Paella	2.5 %
	British Classics Chicken & Bacon Pie	2.5 %
	British Classics Chicken & Mushroom Hotpot	2.5 %
	Big Night In Indian Chicken Korma & Pilau Rice	2.6 %
	Cheese & Onion Quiche	2.6 %
	Classic Italian Tomato & Mozzarella Pasta Bake	2.6 %
	Finest Mapye Cured Bacon & Gruyere Small Quiche	2.6 %
	Finest Red Thai Duck Noodles	2.6 %
	Indian Chicken Jalfrezi and Pilau Rice	2.6 %
	Indian Chicken Tikka Masala & Lamb Rogan Josh Meal For 2	2.6 %
	Indian Lamb Rogan Josh and Pilau Rice	2.6 %
	Modern Italian Fajita Chicken Pasta	2.6 %
	Indian Prawn Masala and Pilau Rice	2.6 %
	Al Fresco King Prawn & Orzo Pasta	2.7 %
	Classic Italian Chicken Lasagne	2.7 %

Ready Meals - by brand (continued)

Brand	Label	% Sugar
Tesco	Everyday Value Chicken Korma And Rice	2.7 %
	Family Favourites Chicken & Tomato Pasta Bake	2.7 %
	Finest Creamy Fish Pie	2.7 %
	Healthy Living Chicken Tikka Masala & Rice	2.7 %
	Healthy Living Sausage & Root Veg Mash	2.7 %
	Indian Chicken Tikka Masala and Pilau Rice	2.7 %
	Modern Italian Chicken Arrabbiata Pasta	2.7 %
	Modern Italian Pepperoni Pasta Bake	2.7 %
	Takeaway Indian Chicken Korma with Pilau Rice & Naan Bread	2.7 %
	Oriental Kung Po Chicken with Egg Fried Rice	2.8 %
	Chicken Jalfrezi	2.8 %
	Chinese Beef & Black Bean Sauce	2.8 %
	Family Favourites Lasagne	2.8 %
	Finest Beef Madras with Pilau Rice	2.8 %
	Finest Hot Piri Piri Chicken and Rice	2.8 %
	Indian Chicken Tikka Masala & Jalfrezi Meal For 2	2.8 %
	Thai Chicken Red Curry with Jasmine Rice	2.8 %
	Big Night In Indian Vegetable Balti & Pilau Rice	2.9 %
	Classic Italian Meatball Pasta Bake	2.9 %
	Everyday Value Chicken Tikka And Rice	2.9 %
	Finest Bourbon Pulled Beef & Sweet Onion Mash	2.9 %
	Cheese & Tomato Quiche	3.0 %
	Classic Italian Sausage Pasta Bake	3.0 %
	Healthy Living Broccoli & Tomato Crustless Quiche	3.0 %
	Sweet Potato & Goat's Cheese Lattice Pie	3.0 %

Ready Meals - by brand (continued)

Brand	Label	% Sugar
Tesco	Al Fresco Spanish Pork & Chorizo Meatballs in Tomato Sauce	3.0 %
	Oriental Chinese Chicken Curry with Egg Fried Rice	3.0 %
	Oriental Meal For 2 Menu C	3.0 %
The City Kitchen	Skinny Thai Coconut Chicken	1.1 %
	Malaysian Coconut Beef Curry	1.5 %
	Malaysian Chicken Curry Noodles	1.7 %
	Vegetables with Coconut & Lentil Pilaf	1.8 %
	Skinny Bombay Spiced Chicken	1.9 %
	Takeaway No 65 Singapore Noodles	1.9 %
	Katsu Chicken Curry	2.5 %
	Thai Chicken Fried Rice	2.5 %
	King Prawn Red Thai Curry	2.8 %
	Indonesian Pulled Pork & Mushroom Noodles	2.9 %
	Chilli Moonshine Beef	2.9 %
Toscana	Mushroom Risotto	0.2 %
	Vegetable Risotto	0.9 %
	Penne Carbonara	1.2 %
	Penne Beef Bolognese	2.3 %
	Penne Tomato & Basil	3.0 %
	Penne Tomato & Chilli	3.0 %
Uncle Ben's	Chicken & Mushroom Risotto	1.0 %
	Bacon & Mushroom Risotto	1.2 %
	Rice Time Spicy Tikka Masala	2.3 %
	Rice Time Medium Curry	2.7 %
	Rice Time Mexican Chilli	2.8 %

Ready Meals - by brand (continued)

Brand	Label	% Sugar
UpperCrust	Deep Filled Steak Pie	0.7 %
	Deep Filled Chicken & Asparagus Pie	0.8 %
Waitrose	Spaghetti Bolognese	0.1 %
	Mushroom Risotto	0.2 %
	Menu Fish Pie	0.3 %
	Beef Stroganoff	0.4 %
	Chicken in Red Wine	0.4 %
	Heston Slow-Cooked Pork	0.4 %
	Frozen Mini Cottage Pie	0.5 %
	Love Life Fish Pie	0.5 %
	Braised Beef and Mash	0.6 %
	Fisherman's Pie	0.6 %
	Heston Fish Pie	0.6 %
	Menu Chicken Tarragon	0.6 %
	Oriental Egg Fried Rice	0.6 %
	Heston Cauliflower Macaroni Cheese	0.7 %
	Menu Mushroom Risotto	0.7 %
	Cottage Pie	0.8 %
	Love Life Beef Fettuccine	0.8 %
	Menu Chicken & Asparagus Risotto	0.8 %
	Oriental Special Fried Rice	0.8 %
	Beef Goulash	0.9 %
	Love Life Cottage Pie	0.9 %
	Spaghetti Carbonara	0.9 %
	Frozen Mini Macaroni Cheese	1.0 %
	Love Life Beef & Red Wine Casserole	1.0 %

Ready Meals - by brand (continued)

Brand	Label	% Sugar
Waitrose	Spicy Fusilli with Sausage	1.0 %
	Chicken Forestiere	1.1 %
	Cumberland Pie	1.1 %
	Macaroni Cheese	1.1 %
	Mushroom and Spinach Linguine	1.1 %
	Bacon & Pea Risotto	1.2 %
	Chicken with Cheese and Bacon	1.2 %
	Frozen Chicken & King Prawn Paella	1.2 %
	Frozen Green Thai Chicken Noodles	1.2 %
	Frozen Mini Sausage & Mash	1.2 %
	Love Life Cod in Parsley Sauce	1.2 %
	Love Life Creamy Chicken & Vegetable Hotpot	1.2 %
	Love Life Ham Hock in Mustard Sauce	1.2 %
	Love Life Red Thai Chicken Curry	1.2 %
	Menu Chicken Forestiere	1.2 %
	Menu Paella	1.2 %
	Shepherd's Pie	1.2 %
	Chicken Hotpot	1.3 %
	Chicken, White Wine & Tarragon Top Crust Pie	1.3 %
	Indian Spinach and Carrot Pilau Rice	1.3 %
	Menu Beef Gratin	1.3 %
	Tagliatelle with Ham	1.3 %
	Bubble & Squeak	1.4 %
	Crustless Spinach, Feta and Roasted Red Pepper Quiche	1.4 %
	Love Life Green Thai Chicken Curry	1.4 %

Ready Meals - by brand (continued)

Brand	Label	% Sugar
Waitrose	Love Life Piri Piri Chicken	1.4 %
	Menu Cottage Pie	1.4 %
	Roast Chicken Large Pie	1.4 %
	Frozen Chicken Biryani	1.5 %
	Frozen Mini Liver & Bacon	1.5 %
	Vegetable Chilli with Rice	1.5 %
	Chicken Tagliatelle	1.6 %
	Chicken, Leek & White Wine Large Pie	1.6 %
	Filled Jacket Potatoes	1.6 %
	Indian Spinach Dal	1.6 %
	Love Life Pea & Spinach Open Ravioli	1.6 %
	Menu Beef Stroganoff	1.6 %
	Menu Ham Hock & Camembert Crepes	1.6 %
	Spinach Mornay	1.6 %
	Menu Quiche Lorraine	1.7 %
	Menu Smoked Fish Gratin	1.7 %
	Steak Large Pie	1.7 %
	Chicken & Chorizo Paella	1.8 %
	Chicken Pie	1.8 %
	Chicken Provençal	1.8 %
	Cod Fillet in Parsley Sauce	1.8 %
	Delisante Artisan Salmon & Watercress Quiche	1.8 %
	Frozen Roast Chicken Pies	1.8 %
	Garlic Mushroom Gratin	1.8 %
	Indian Tarka Dahl	1.8 %
	Love Life Roasted Mushroom Risotto	1.8 %

Ready Meals - by brand (continued)

Brand	Label	% Sugar
Waitrose	Orkney Crab Gratin	1.8 %
	Spinach Cannelloni	1.8 %
	Cajun Chicken Tagliatelle	1.9 %
	Menu Shepherd's Pie	1.9 %
	Piri Piri Chicken	1.9 %
	Quiche Lorraine	1.9 %
	Rigatoni and Aubergine	1.9 %
	Steak & Stout Pie	1.9 %
	Broccoli & Gruyère Quiche	2.0 %
	Chicken, Ham Hock & Leek Pie	2.0 %
	Frozen Mini Chicken Dinner	2.0 %
	Frozen Seafood Risotto	2.0 %
	Frozen Steak & Ale Pies	2.0 %
	Ham Hock in Cider & Mustard Sauce	2.0 %
	Love Life Harissa Chicken	2.0 %
	Love Life Smoky Chorizo Chicken	2.0 %
	Menu Mushroom Open Ravioli	2.0 %
	Steak & Kidney Puddings	2.0 %
	Frozen Mini Spaghetti Bolognese	2.1 %
	Frozen Steak & Mushroom Pies	2.1 %
	Lamb Hotpot	2.1 %
	Quiche Lorraine Small	2.1 %
	Steak, Mushroom & Red Wine Pie	2.1 %
	Love Life Spinach & Ricotta Cannelloni	2.2 %
	Menu Beef Bourguignon	2.2 %
	Yorkshire with Sausage and Mash	2.2 %

Ready Meals - by brand (continued)

Brand	Label	% Sugar
Waitrose	Beef Casserole	2.3 %
	Essential Bacon, Leek & Cheddar Cheese Quiche	2.3 %
	Frozen Vegetarian Cottage Pie	2.3 %
	Haddock in Cheese Sauce	2.3 %
	Love Life Lasagne	2.3 %
	Quiche Lorraine Crustless	2.3 %
	Roast Chicken Pie	2.3 %
	Steak Pie	2.3 %
	Braised Steak, Portobello Mushroom & Red Wine Pie	2.4 %
	Chilli con Carne with Rice	2.4 %
	Heston Chilli Con Carne	2.4 %
	Indian Chicken Shashlik	2.4 %
	Liver and Bacon	2.4 %
	Love Life Beef & Barbecue Beans	2.4 %
	Love Life Butternut Squash Risotto	2.4 %
	Oriental Chicken Chow Mein	2.4 %
	Roasted Red Pepper Goats Cheese Quiche	2.4 %
	Vintage Cheddar & Onion Small Quiche	2.4 %
	Bacon, Leek & Roquefort Tart	2.5 %
	Beef Cannelloni	2.5 %
	Delisante Artisan Quiche Lorraine	2.5 %
	Essential Cheddar Cheese & Onion Quiche	2.5 %
	Frozen Pea & Asparagus Risotto	2.5 %
	Indian Goan Fish Curry	2.5 %
	Indian Vegetable Thoran	2.5 %
	Love Life Chicken Kastu Curry & Jasmine Rice	2.5 %

Ready Meals - by brand (continued)

Brand	Label	% Sugar
Waitrose	Love Life Spicy Jerk Chicken	2.5 %
	Spinach & Ricotta Quiche	2.5 %
	Beef Lasagne	2.6 %
	Chicken Enchiladas	2.6 %
	Love Life Chicken Korma with Pilau Rice	2.6 %
	Love Life Tomato & Rosemary Chicken	2.6 %
	Mushroom & Spinach Filo Parcel	2.6 %
	Roast Beef Dinner	2.6 %
	Rosemary Chicken Penne	2.6 %
	Vintage Cheddar & Onion Quiche	2.6 %
	Chicken Arrabiata	2.7 %
	Frozen Mini Lasagne	2.7 %
	Frozen Vegetarian Chestnuts & Mushroom Grills	2.7 %
	Menu Beef Lasagne	2.7 %
	Leek Gratin	2.8 %
	Love Life Beef & Pork Meatballs with Spaghetti	2.8 %
	Love Life Chicken & Prawn Paella	2.8 %
	Menu Beef Casserole	2.8 %
	Frozen Vegetarian Goats Cheese & Spinach Slices	2.9 %
	Indian Aloo Gobi Saag	2.9 %
	Love Life Lamb Moussaka	2.9 %
	Love Life Roasted Vegetable Lasagne	2.9 %
	Four Cheese Ravioli	3.0 %
	Frozen Vegetarian Lasagne	3.0 %
	Indian Lamb Kofta Curry	3.0 %

Ready Meals - by brand (continued)

Brand	Label	% Sugar
Weight Watchers	Chicken & Mushroom Pie	0.7 %
	Chicken Korma with Basmati Rice	1.1 %
	Red Thai Curry with Jasmine Rice	1.1 %
	Chicken, Tomato & Spinach Lasagne	1.3 %
	Classic Cottage Pie	1.3 %
	Chicken Tikka with Basmati Rice	1.4 %
	Spanish Chicken & Patatas Bravas	1.5 %
	Cheese & Onion Crustless Quiche	1.7 %
	Macaroni Cheese	1.7 %
	Chicken Jambalaya	1.8 %
	Bacon & Leek Crustless Quiche	2.2 %
	Lincolnshire Sausages & Mash	2.4 %
	Bolognese al Forno	2.5 %
	Jamaican Jerk Chicken Curry with Rice	2.5 %
	Hunters Chicken with Brown & Wild Rice	2.6 %
	Szechuan Chicken with Rice	2.7 %
Weight Watchers From Heinz	Chicken Curry	0.6 %
	Chicken & Lemon Risotto	0.8 %
	Chicken & Mushroom Tagliatelle	0.8 %
	Beef Lasagne	1.2 %
	Cottage Pie	1.4 %
	Beef Hotpot	1.7 %
	Chicken In White Wine Sauce	1.7 %
	Ocean Pie	1.9 %

Ready Meals - by brand (continued)

Brand	Label	% Sugar
Weight Watchers From Heinz	Spaghetti Bolognese	2.0 %
	Thai Green Chicken Curry	2.0 %
	Salmon & Broccoli Wedge Melt	2.3 %
	Mexican Chilli	2.5 %
	Chicken Hotpot	2.6 %
Young's	Chip Shop Fish Steak & Chips	0.6 %
	Fish Fillet Quarter Pounder & Chips	0.7 %
	Gastro Cod Spinach, Cheese & Potato Gratin	0.7 %
	Scampi Bites & Chips	0.8 %
	Gastro Gratin Dauphinoise Fish Pie	0.9 %
	Chip Shop Large Cod Fillet & Chips	1.0 %
	Gastro Pink Salmon, Alaska Pollock & Cherry Tomato Bake	1.3 %
	Admiral's Pie	1.9 %
	Fisherman's Pie	2.0 %
	Ocean Pie	2.0 %
	Salmon Crumble	2.2 %
	Fish Fillet Dinner	2.3 %
	Low Fat Ocean Crumble	2.5 %
	Salmon Fillet Dinner	2.6 %
	Mariner's Pie	2.8 %

Fast Food

Supermarkets aren't the only place you'll be buying food prepared by others. To cover off the majority of the market for 'restaurant' food, in this section, I've analysed the menus of the major fast food chains.

> **WARNING:** All fried food sold in these restaurants in Britain has been fried in seed oils and should be avoided if you are concerned about seed oils.

Subway Restaurants

Category	Item	% Sugar
Breakfast Flatbreads	Mega Melt	1.8 %
	Bacon	1.8 %
	Bacon, Egg & Cheese	1.8 %
	Sausage, Egg & Cheese	1.9 %
	Egg & Cheese	2.0 %
	Sausage	2.0 %
Breakfast Subs 9-grain Bread	Mega Melt	2.3 %
	Sausage, Egg & Cheese	2.5 %
	Bacon, Egg & Cheese	2.7 %
	Sausage	2.8 %
	Bacon	2.8 %
	Egg & Cheese	3.0 %
Breakfast Subs Italian Bread	Bacon, Egg & Cheese	2.9 %
	Egg & Cheese	2.0 %
Flatbread Sandwiches	Chicken & Bacon Ranch Melt	1.4 %
	Chicken Temptation	1.6 %

Subway Restaurants (continued)

Category	Item	% Sugar
Flatbread Sandwiches	Tuna	1.6 %
	Spicy Italian	1.8 %
	Italian BMT	1.9 %
	Steak & Cheese	1.9 %
	Subway Melt	1.9 %
	Big Beef Melt	2.0 %
	Veggie Patty	2.7 %
Kids Pak Subs 9-grain Bread	Beef	2.5 %
	Ham	2.8 %
	Turkey Breast	2.5 %
Kids Pak Subs Italian Bread	Beef	2.8 %
	Turkey Breast	2.8 %
Low Fat Flatbread Sandwiches	Chicken Teriyaki	2.7 %
	Chicken Breast	1.7 %
	Beef	1.8 %
	Chicken Tikka	2.5 %
	Turkey Breast & Ham	1.8 %
	Subway Club	1.7 %
	Turkey Breast	1.8 %
	Ham	2.0 %
	Veggie Delite	2.2 %
	Tandoori Chicken	2.0 %
Low Fat Subs 9-grain Bread	Subway Club	2.1 %
	Chicken Breast	2.2 %
	Beef	2.3 %
	Turkey Breast	2.3 %

Subway Restaurants (continued)

Category	Item	% Sugar
Low Fat Subs 9-grain Bread	Turkey Breast & Ham	2.4 %
	Tandoori Chicken	2.5 %
	Ham	2.6 %
	Chicken Tikka	2.9 %
	Veggie Delite	3.0 %
Low Fat Subs Italian Bread	Subway Club	2.6 %
	Chicken Breast	2.7 %
	Beef	2.8 %
	Turkey Breast	2.8 %
	Turkey Breast & Ham	2.9 %
	Chicken Tikka	2.9 %
	Veggie Delite	3.0 %
Regular Subs 9-grain Bread	Chicken & Bacon Ranch Melt	1.9 %
	Chicken Temptation	2.0 %
	Tuna	2.2 %
	Spicy Italian	2.3 %
	Subway Melt	2.4 %
	Italian BMT	2.4 %
	Steak & Cheese	2.7 %
	Big Beef Melt	3.0 %
Regular Subs Italian Bread	Chicken & Bacon Ranch Melt	2.2 %
	Chicken Temptation	2.4 %
	Tuna	2.7 %
	Spicy Italian	2.8 %
	Subway Melt	2.9 %
	Italian BMT	2.9 %

Subway Restaurants (continued)

Category	Item	% Sugar
Regular Subs Italian Bread	Veggie Patty	2.9 %
	Big Beef Melt	3.0 %
Salads	Subway Club	1.3 %
	Chicken Breast	1.4 %
	Beef	1.4 %
	Turkey Breast	1.4 %
	Turkey Breast & Ham	1.4 %
	Chicken Tikka	1.5 %
	Ham	1.5 %
	Veggie Delite	1.6 %
	Chicken Teriyaki	2.1 %
Sides & Snacks	Garden Side Salad	1.6 %
	Melted Cheese Nachos	2.3 %
Soup	Cream of Chicken	0.1 %
	Minestrone	0.2 %
	Highland Vegetable	0.3 %
	Country Chicken & Vegetable	0.4 %
	Wild Mushroom	0.5 %
	Lentil & Bacon	0.8 %
	Cream of Mushroom	0.9 %
	Beef Goulash	1.8 %
	Carrot & Coriander	2.4 %
	Leek & Potato	2.5 %
	Tomato	2.5 %

McDonald's

McDonald's in the UK no longer publish nutrition information in a format which allows easy comparison (per 100g). So this table uses the amount of sugar per portion (for example – 1 burger). If an item contains more than 3g of sugar it has been excluded from this list.

All McDonald's fried food in the UK is fried in a Sunflower and Rapeseed oil blend. If you are avoiding seed oils then you should avoid anything on this list which is fried.

Product Type	Item	Grams per portion
Chicken	Crispy Chicken Salad	3.0 g
	Crispy Chicken & Bacon Salad	3.0 g
	ShareBox® - 5 Chicken McNugget portion	0.5 g
	20 Chicken McNuggets® ShareBox®	1.9 g
	Chicken McNuggets® (4 pieces)	0.4 g
	Chicken McNuggets® (6 pieces)	0.6 g
	Chicken McNuggets® (9 pieces)	0.8 g
	Chicken Selects® (3 pieces)	0.3 g
	Chicken Selects® (5 pieces)	0.5 g
Fish	Fish Fingers	0.5 g
Salad	Shaker Side Salad	1.9 g
Sides	Cheese Bites	0.8 g
	French Fries Small	0.4 g
	French Fries Medium	0.6 g
	French Fries Large	0.8 g
	Hash Brown	0.3 g
Breakfast	All unflavoured and unsweetened Tea and Coffee*	0.0 g

McDonald's (continued)

Product Type	Item	Grams per portion
Breakfast	McMuffin® with Egg	2.1 g
	Double Bacon & Egg McMuffin®	2.2 g
	Bacon & Egg McMuffin®	2.1 g
	Sausage & Egg McMuffin®	2.7 g
Little Tasters	Spicy Mayo Snack Wrap®	1.8 g

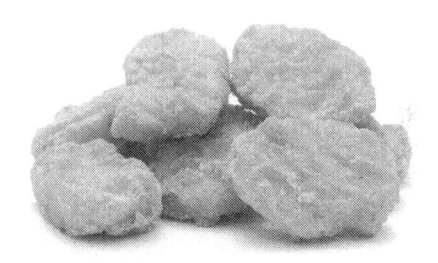

Burger King

The sugar content of most menu items at Burger King is surprisingly high in Britain. The only items that qualify are listed below.

Category	Item	% Sugar
Beef & Chicken	Chicken Royale	2.9 %
	Chicken Royale with Cheese	3.0 %
	Tendercrisp	2.4 %
	Tendercrisp with Cheese	2.5 %
	BLT Chicken Wrap	2.0 %
Sides	Fries	0.2 %
	Chilli Cheese Bites	1.4 %
Veggie, Fish & Salad	King Fish	2.3 %
Breakfast	Hash Browns	0.0 %
Extras	Whopper Patty	0.0 %
	Angus Patty	0.0 %
	Hamburger Patty	0.0 %
	Pork Sausage Breakfast Patty	0.2 %
	Egg Patty	1.2 %
	Pickles	0.0 %
	Lettuce	2.1 %
	Pepperjack Cheese Slice	2.4 %
	Edam Cheese Slice	0.0 %

Pizza Hut

Pizza Hut in the UK no longer publish nutrition information for their pizzas in a format which allows easy comparison (per 100g). So the pizza table uses the amount of sugar per slice. If a slice contains more than 3g of sugar it has been excluded from this list.

Note: These figures have not been adjusted for lactose (in the cheese) content as it is difficult to accurately estimate. All figures would be lower when adjusted for lactose.

Type	Size	Grams per slice
Veggie	Individual Pan (9")	1.9 g
	Individual Thin (11")	1.3 g
	Large Thin (14")	2.2 g
	Individual Ultimate Thin (11")	1.4 g
	Large Ultimate Thin (14")	2.3 g
	Individual Stuffed Crust (11")	1.4 g
	Large Stuffed Crust (14")	2.3 g
	Cheesy Bites (14")	2.3 g
	Gluten Free (9" Square)	1.8 g
Pepperoni Feast	Individual Pan (9")	1.4 g
	Large Pan (13")	2.1 g
	Individual Thin (11")	0.9 g
	Large Thin (14")	1.3 g
	Individual Ultimate Thin (11")	0.9 g
	Large Ultimate Thin (14")	1.4 g
	Individual Stuffed Crust (11")	0.9 g
	Large Stuffed Crust (14")	1.3 g
	Cheesy Bites (14")	1.3 g

Pizza Hut (continued)

Type	Size	Grams per slice
Pepperoni Feast	Gluten Free (9" Square)	1.3 g
Veggie Hot One	Individual Pan (9")	1.9 g
	Large Pan (13")	3.0 g
	Individual Thin (11")	1.3 g
	Large Thin (14")	2.1 g
	Individual Ultimate Thin (11")	1.4 g
	Large Ultimate Thin (14")	2.2 g
	Individual Stuffed Crust (11")	1.4 g
	Large Stuffed Crust (14")	2.2 g
	Cheesy Bites (14")	2.2 g
	Gluten Free (9" Square)	1.8 g
Chicken Supreme	Individual Pan (9")	2.7 g
	Individual Thin (11")	2.2 g
	Individual Ultimate Thin (11")	2.6 g
	Individual Stuffed Crust (11")	2.2 g
	Gluten Free (9" Square)	2.6 g
Margherita	Individual Pan (9")	1.5 g
	Large Pan (13")	2.3 g
	Individual Thin (11")	1.0 g
	Large Thin (14")	1.4 g
	Individual Ultimate Thin (11")	1.0 g
	Large Ultimate Thin (14")	1.5 g
	Individual Stuffed Crust (11")	1.0 g
	Large Stuffed Crust (14")	1.5 g
	Cheesy Bites (14")	1.5 g
	Gluten Free (9" Square)	1.4 g

Pizza Hut (continued)

Type	Size	Grams per slice
Meat Feast	Individual Pan (9")	1.5 g
	Large Pan (13")	2.4 g
	Individual Thin (11")	1.0 g
	Large Thin (14")	1.5 g
	Individual Ultimate Thin (11")	1.1 g
	Large Ultimate Thin (14")	1.6 g
	Individual Stuffed Crust (11")	1.1 g
	Large Stuffed Crust (14")	1.6 g
	Cheesy Bites (14")	1.6 g
	Gluten Free (9" Square)	1.4 g
BBQ Meat Feast	Individual Thin (11")	2.8 g
	Individual Ultimate Thin (11")	1.9 g
	Large Ultimate Thin (14")	2.9 g
	Individual Stuffed Crust (11")	2.8 g
Supreme	Individual Pan (9")	1.8 g
	Large Pan (13")	2.8 g
	Individual Thin (11")	1.3 g
	Large Thin (14")	2.0 g
	Individual Ultimate Thin (11")	1.3 g
	Large Ultimate Thin (14")	2.0 g
	Individual Stuffed Crust (11")	1.3 g
	Large Stuffed Crust (14")	2.0 g
	Cheesy Bites (14")	2.0 g
	Gluten Free (9" Square)	1.7 g
BBQ Americano	Individual Thin (11")	2.9 g
	Individual Ultimate Thin (11")	3.0 g

Pizza Hut (continued)

Type	Size	Grams per slice
BBQ Americano	Individual Stuffed Crust (11")	3.0 g
Hawaiian	Individual Pan (9")	2.2 g
	Individual Thin (11")	1.7 g
	Large Thin (14")	2.7 g
	Individual Ultimate Thin (11")	1.8 g
	Large Ultimate Thin (14")	2.8 g
	Individual Stuffed Crust (11")	1.7 g
	Large Stuffed Crust (14")	2.8 g
	Cheesy Bites (14")	2.8 g
	Gluten Free (9" Square)	2.1 g
New Orleans Cajun Chicken	Individual Pan (9")	2.5 g
	Individual Thin (11")	2.0 g
	Individual Ultimate Thin (11")	2.1 g
	Large Ultimate Thin (14")	2.0 g
	Gluten Free (9" Square)	2.4 g
Blazin' Inferno	Individual Pan (9")	1.8 g
	Large Pan (13")	2.9 g
	Individual Thin (11")	1.3 g
	Large Thin (14")	2.0 g
	Individual Ultimate Thin (11")	1.4 g
	Large Ultimate Thin (14")	2.1 g
	Individual Stuffed Crust (11")	1.3 g
	Large Stuffed Crust (14")	2.1 g
	Cheesy Bites (14")	2.1 g
	Gluten Free (9" Square)	1.7 g

Pizza Hut (continued)

Type	Size	Grams per slice
Heavenly Veg	Individual Pan (9")	2.8 g
	Individual Thin (11")	2.3 g
	Individual Stuffed Crust (11")	2.3 g
	Gluten Free (9" Square)	2.7 g
Phillycheese Steak	Individual Pan (9")	2.7 g
	Individual Thin (11")	2.2 g
	Large Thin (14")	2.4 g
	Individual Ultimate Thin (11")	2.7 g
	Individual Stuffed Crust (11")	2.2 g
	Large Stuffed Crust (14")	2.4 g
	Cheesy Bites (14")	2.4 g
	Gluten Free (9" Square)	2.6 g
King of the Coast	Individual Pan (9")	1.2 g
	Large Pan (13")	1.8 g
	Individual Thin (11")	0.6 g
	Large Thin (14")	0.9 g
	Individual Ultimate Thin (11")	0.7 g
	Large Ultimate Thin (14")	1.0 g
	Individual Stuffed Crust (11")	0.7 g
	Large Stuffed Crust (14")	1.0 g
	Cheesy Bites (14")	1.0 g
	Gluten Free (9" Square)	1.1 g
Texas Meat Meltdown	Individual Thin (11")	2.8 g
	Individual Ultimate Thin (11")	3.0 g
	Individual Stuffed Crust (11")	2.8 g

Pizza Hut (continued)

Type	Size	Grams per slice
Beef Fajita	Individual Pan (9")	2.9 g
	Individual Thin (11")	2.4 g
	Individual Ultimate Thin (11")	2.3 g
	Individual Stuffed Crust (11")	2.5 g
	Gluten Free (9" Square)	2.8 g
500 Cal Pizza	Shrimply Delicious	1.0 g
	Chicken Delight	0.9 g
	Virtuous Veg	0.9 g
	HAPPY HOUR	
Margherita	Individual Pan (9")	1.5 g
	Individual Thin (11")	1.0 g
Ham & Sweetcorn	Individual Pan (9")	1.6 g
	Individual Thin (11")	1.1 g
Pepperoni & Jalapeno	Individual Pan (9")	1.4 g
	Individual Thin (11")	0.9 g
Pepperoni	Individual Pan (9")	1.4 g
	Individual Thin (11")	0.9 g
	Individual Pan (9")	1.6 g
Mushroom & Onion	Individual Thin (11")	1.0 g
Chicken & Onion	Individual Pan (9")	1.6 g
	Individual Thin (11")	1.1 g
	BUFFET	
Margherita	Individual Pan (9")	1.1 g
	Large Pan (13")	1.8 g
	Individual Thin (11")	0.7 g
	Large Thin (14")	1.1 g

Pizza Hut (continued)

Type	Size	Grams per slice
Hawaiian	Individual Pan (9")	1.7 g
	Large Pan (13")	2.9 g
	Individual Thin (11")	1.3 g
	Large Thin (14")	2.2 g
Pepperoni Feast	Individual Pan (9")	1.0 g
	Large Pan (13")	1.7 g
	Individual Thin (11")	0.7 g
	Large Thin (14")	1.0 g
Chicken Supreme	Individual Pan (9")	2.0 g
	Individual Thin (11")	1.6 g
	Large Thin (14")	2.8 g
Veggie Hot One	Individual Pan (9")	1.4 g
	Large Pan (13")	2.4 g
	Individual Thin (11")	1.0 g
	Large Thin (14")	1.7 g
BBQ Americano	Individual Pan (9")	2.6 g
	Individual Thin (11")	2.2 g
BBQ Beef & Onion	Individual Pan (9")	2.8 g
	Individual Thin (11")	2.4 g
Cheese & Caramelised Onion	Individual Pan (9")	2.0 g
	Individual Thin (11")	1.6 g
	Large Thin (14")	2.8 g
Veggie	Individual Pan (9")	1.4 g
	Large Pan (13")	2.4 g
	Individual Thin (11")	1.0 g

Pizza Hut (continued)

Type	Size	Grams per slice
Veggie	Large Thin (14")	1.8 g
Chorizo & Jalapeno	Individual Pan (9")	1.0 g
	Large Pan (13")	1.7 g
	Individual Thin (11")	0.6 g
	Large Thin (14")	1.0 g
Ham & Mushroom	Individual Pan (9")	1.1 g
	Large Pan (13")	1.8 g
	Individual Thin (11")	0.7 g
	Large Thin (14")	1.1 g
Cajun Chicken & Roquito® Peppers	Individual Pan (9")	1.7 g
	Large Pan (13")	2.9 g
	Individual Thin (11")	1.3 g
	Large Thin (14")	2.2 g

Oddly Pizza Hut do prepare a list calculated per 100g for all their sides, dips, pastas and Kids' Pizzas so here are the items from that list that comply (in the more standard percentage format)

Category	Item	% Sugar
Starters	Ultimate Garlic Bread	2.8%
	Bruschetta Garlic Bread	2.6%
	Breaded Chicken Strips	0.7%
	Potato Wedges	1.0%
	Alabama Popcorn Shrimp	1.0%
	Cheese Triangles	1.1%
	Cheesy Nachos	2.7%

Pizza Hut (continued)

Category	Item	% Sugar
Starters	Favourites Platter	1.5%
Dips	Sour Cream & Chive Sauce	0.6%
	Mustard Mayo	2.0%
Pastas	Salmon Pasta Bake	1.4%
	Chicken Herby Pasta Bake	1.3%
	4 Cheese Pasta	2.2%
	Bolognese Pasta	3.0%
Salads	Cheesy Sweetcorn Pasta	1.6%
Dried Items	Bacon Bits	1.8%
	Large Salad Croutons	1.1%
	Tortilla Chips	1.6%
	Breadsticks	1.5%
Kids	Smiley Face Margherita Thick Pan Pizza	2.2%
	Smiley Face Ham Thick Pan Pizza	2.1%
	Smiley Face Pepperoni Thick Pan Pizza	2.1%
	Cheesy Macaroni	2.1%
	Ham & Cheesy Pasta	2.0%
	New Kids Spaghetti Bolognese	2.8%

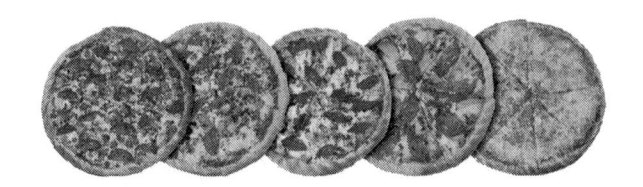

Domino's Pizza

There are no pizzas which qualify at Domino's in the UK. The sugar content ranges from 3.2% (Pepperoni Passion Double Decadence) to 16.9% (Italian Style BBQ Chicken Melt).

Category	Item	% Sugar
Side Orders	Chicken Kickers	0.9 %
	Chicken Strippers	0.4 %
	Chicken Wings	1.5 %
	Frank's RedHot Wings	0.2 %
	Nachos	2.0 %
	Nachos without Jalapenos	2.2 %
	Fajita Potato Wedges	1.0 %
	Potato Wedges	1.0 %
	Garlic & Herb Dip	1.7 %

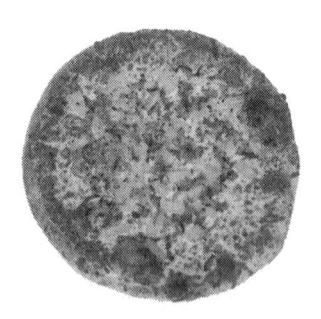

KFC

KFC in the UK no longer publish nutrition information in a format which allows easy comparison (per 100g). So this table uses the amount of sugar per portion (for example - 1 piece). If an item contains more than 3g of sugar it has been excluded from this list.

Type	Item	Grams per serve
Original Recipe Chicken	Keel	0.4 g
	Drumstick	0.2 g
	Thigh	0.3 g
	Rib	0.4 g
	Wing	0.3 g
Chicken Burgers	Kids	1.8 g
Twisters & Salads	Streetwise® Wraps - Flamin'	2.9 g
Chicken Pieces	Popcorn Chicken® - Kids/Small	0.3 g
	Popcorn Chicken® - Regular	0.6 g
	Popcorn Chicken® - Large	1.0 g
	Hot Wings®	0.1 g
	Mini Breast Fillets / Boneless Dips	0.3 g
Sides	Fries - Regular	0.4 g
	Fries - Large	0.6 g
	Corn Cobette - Regular	1.9 g
	Gravy - Regular	0.9 g
	Gravy - Large	2.0 g
Drinks	Water - 500ml bottle	0.0 g
	Robinsons® Fruit Shoots	1.6 g
	Pepsi Max/Diet Pepsi/Diet Coke/Coke Zero (Kids, Regular, Large), 7Up free	0.0 g
	Usweetened, unflavoured Tea & Coffee	0.0 g

Pret a Manger

Category	Item	% Sugar
Soups	Aromatic Asian Chicken Soup	1.6 %
	Chicken & Ham Soup	0.8 %
	Chicken, Broccoli & Brown Rice Soup	1.0 %
	Chicken, Edamame & Ginger Soup	1.5 %
	Cream of Chicken Soup	1.8 %
	Mushroom Risotto Soup	0.9 %
	Sag Aloo Soup	1.4 %
	South Indian Tomato & Spice Soup	2.5 %
	Thai Chicken Curry Soup	1.9 %
	Thai Corn Soup	0.6 %
	Tuscan Minestrone Soup	1.6 %
Sandwiches	All Day Breakfast	3.0 %
	Beech Smoked BLT	2.7 %
	Chicken Avocado	1.9 %
	Classic Super Club	2.2 %
	Cracking Egg Salad	2.2 %
	Egg & Tomato on Rye	2.1 %
	Free-Range Egg Mayo	1.8 %
	Kid's Cheese Sandwich	2.5 %
	Kid's Ham Sandwich	2.6 %
	Pole & Line Caught Tuna & Rocket	1.8 %
	Scottish Smoked Salmon	2.0 %
	Super Greens Sandwich	2.6 %
	Wild Crayfish & Rocket	1.9 %
Baguettes	Brie, Tomato & Basil Baguette	2.1 %
	Chicken Caesar & Bacon on Artisan	1.9 %

Pret a Manger (continued)

Category	Item	% Sugar
Baguettes	Classic Ham & Eggs	1.5 %
	Italian Prosciutto on Artisan	2.2 %
	Jambon-Beurre	1.4 %
	Mini French Baguette	2.5 %
	Pole & Line Caught Tuna Mayo & Cucumber Baguette	1.3 %
	Wiltshire-Cured Ham & Greve Cheese Baguette	1.6 %
Wraps	Avocado & Chipotle Chicken Flatbread	1.5 %
	Avocado & Herb Salad Wrap	1.9 %
	Chicken Raita Salad Wrap	2.7 %
	Chunky Humous Salad Wrap	2.0 %
	Mediterranean Tuna Flat Bread	2.5 %
	Roasted Salmon & Avocado	2.7 %
Pret's Hot	Brie, Tomato & Basil Toastie	1.9 %
	Chicken & Bacon Toastie	1.2 %
	Halloumi & Red Pepper Toastie	3.0 %
	Ham, Cheese & Mustard Toastie	1.3 %
	Macaroni Cheese Kale & Cauli	1.8 %
	Macaroni Cheese Prosciutto	1.8 %
	Tuna Melt Toastie	1.0 %
Salads	Chef's Chipotle Chicken Salad	1.8 %
	Chef's Italian Chicken Salad	2.1 %
	Chicken & Broccoli Super Noodle Salad	2.4 %
	Crayfish & Quinoa Protein Pot	1.0 %
	Crayfish and Avocado No Bread	0.6 %
	Egg & Spinach Protein Pot	0.3 %

Pret a Manger (continued)

Category	Item	% Sugar
Baguettes	Salmon & Avocado Protein Pot	0.9 %
	Smoked Salmon & Egg Protein Pot	0.3 %
	Superfood Salad	2.2 %
	Tuna Nicoise Salad	1.2 %
Pret Snacks	Maldon Sea Salt Crisps	0.5 %
	Matured Cheddar & Red Onion Crisps	2.3 %
	Rock Salt Popcorn	0.3 %
	Sea Salt & Organic Cider Vinegar Crisps	1.3 %
Sweet Treats	Dairy-free Coconut Yoghurt Pot	2.0 %
Breakfast	British Bacon & Egg Roll	1.4 %
	British Bacon Breakfast Roll	1.4 %
	British Sausage & Egg Roll	2.0 %
	Five Grain Porridge	1.6 %
	Free-Range Egg Mayo & Bacon Breakfast Baguette	2.0 %
	Free-Range Egg Mayo & Roasted Tomato Breakfast Baguette	1.5 %
	Ham & Egg Roll	1.5 %
	Pret's Proper Porridge	2.2 %
	Smoked Salmon & Free Range Egg Breakfast Baguette	1.1 %

EAT

Category	Item	% Sugar
Classic Sandwiches	Cheddar & Pickle	2.7 %
	Crayfish & Rocket	2.4 %
	Ham & Free Range Egg Bloomer	0.8 %
	New York Pastrami Bloomer	0.5 %
	Roast Chicken Salad	2.7 %
	Roast Chicken, Pork, Sage & Onion Bloomer	1.1 %
	Simple Chunky Free Range Egg Mayonnaise and Watercress	1.8 %
	Simple Free Range Egg Mayonnaise and Cress	2.0 %
	Simple Skipjack Tuna, Mayonnaise and Cucumber	2.4 %
	Smoked Chicken, Tomato & Pesto Bloomer	2.2 %
	Smoked Scottish Salmon & Soft Cheese	2.4 %
	Tuna & Rocket	1.4 %
Baguettes	Brie, Tomato and Basil	1.4 %
	Chicken, Avocado & Bacon	1.4 %
	Ham and Jarlsberg	0.6 %
	Houmous & Avocado	1.7 %
	Roast Chicken Salad	1.2 %
	The EAT Club	1.3 %
	Tuna and Cucumber	0.8 %
Wraps	Ham Hock & Cheddar Salad	2.1 %
	Houmous & Falafel	2.5 %
	Simple Roast Chicken	2.2 %

EAT (continued)

Category	Item	% Sugar
Wraps	Thai King Prawn	1.7 %
Toasties	Firecracker Chicken	2.8 %
	Mozzarella, Tomato & Pesto	1.2 %
	Simply Ham and Cheese	0.8 %
	Smoked Chicken and Basil	1.7 %
	Tuna and Cheddar Melt	0.7 %
Hot Flats	Halloumi and Red Pepper Tapenade	2.5 %
Hot Rolls	British Back Bacon	0.7 %
	British Back Bacon & Poached Egg	0.8 %
	Poached Egg, Mushroom & Cheese	1.0 %
	Slow Cooked Beef & Horseradish	1.3 %
Hot Pots	Mac n' Cheese	1.5 %
	Poached Egg, Our Recipe Bean & Ham Hock	2.7 %
	Poached Egg, Our Recipe Bean & Mushrooms	2.9 %
	Poached Egg, Our Recipe Bean with Ham Hock & Mushrooms	2.9 %
	Slow Cooked Beef & Moroccan Vegetable	2.0 %
	Slow Cooked Moroccan Vegetable	2.2 %
	Texan Chilli with Rice	2.1 %
	Thai Green Chicken Curry with Rice	2.7 %
	Vietnamese Chicken Curry	2.8 %
Soups	Bold Hot and Sour Chicken	1.1 %
	Bold Chicken Laksa	0.6 %
	Bold Chicken Pot Pie	1.5 %
	Bold Chicken Tortilla	2.2 %

EAT (continued)

Category	Item	% Sugar
Soups	Bold Coconut Chicken Noodle	1.2 %
	Bold Fully Loaded Potato & Bacon	1.9 %
	Bold Hearty Chicken & Barley	2.3 %
	Bold Hungarian Goulash	1.5 %
	Bold Italian Meatball	2.4 %
	Bold Jerk Chicken	2.2 %
	Bold Salsa Chilli Beef	1.8 %
	Chilli Non Carne	2.7 %
	Chunky Vegetable Minestrone	2.9 %
	Creamy Sweetcorn	3.0 %
	Old Fashioned Chicken & Egg Noodle	1.7 %
	Thai Green Chicken Curry	2.3 %
Noodle Soup Pots	Chicken & Rice Noodles	0.8 %
	Chicken Gyoza Miso	1.2 %
	Duck Gyoza Dumpling & Egg Noodles	2.5 %
	Prawn Tom Yum Pho	1.2 %
	Spicy Rare Beef Noodle	1.5 %
	Vegetable Gyoza Dumpling & Egg Noodles	1.1 %
Bread	Crusty Roll	1.0 %
	Gluten Free Bread Roll	3.0 %
	Seeded Rye Bread	2.1 %
	White Soup Roll	0.4 %
Pies	Beef & Ale Pie	2.9 %
	Cheese & Onion Pie	1.0 %

EAT (continued)

Category	Item	% Sugar
Pies	Chicken & Mushroom Pie	1.5 %
	Chicken, Bacon & Stuffing Pie	2.2 %
	Mature Cheddar & Bacon Quiche	2.4 %
	Roasted Butternut Squash & Feta Pie	2.1 %
	Spinach, Feta & Tomato Quiche	2.3 %
	Steak & Red Wine Pie	1.5 %
Salads	Ham Hock & Egg Side Salad	1.8 %
	Hot Smoked Salmon & Potato	1.6 %
	Houmous Detox Box	2.5 %
	Omega Boosta Salmon Box	1.5 %
	Prawn Cocktail Side Salad	1.9 %
	Simple Chicken Salad	1.7 %
	Simply Tuna Salad	1.8 %
	Supergreens & Feta Side Salad	2.8 %
Breakfast	Cheese & Marmite Toast Melt	0.8 %
	Ham & Cheese Croissant	2.9 %
	Multigrain Toast & Marmite Portion	1.8 %
	Multigrain with Butter	1.8 %

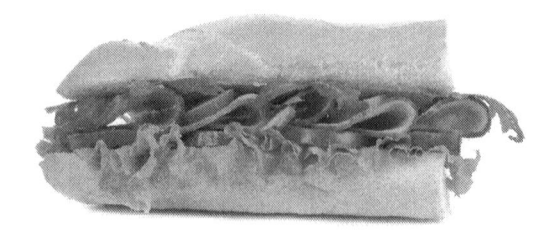

More Information

Still haven't found what you're looking for? I also maintain a database of over 2,000 foods including restaurant meals typically found in Asian and Mediterranean restaurants.

You can search the database for free at www.davidgillespie.org

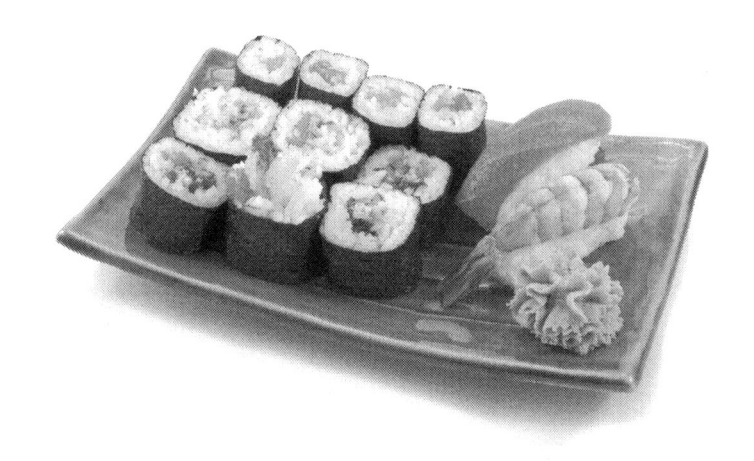

© David Gillespie 2015

The moral right of the author has been asserted. All rights reserved. Without limiting the rights under copyright reserved above, no part of this publication may be reproduced, stored in or introduced into a retrieval system, or transmitted, in any form or by any means (electronic, mechanical, photocopying, recording or otherwise), without the prior written permission of both the copyright owner and the publisher of this book

Published by the Morton Gillespie Pty Ltd
PO Box 196, Cannon Hill QLD 4170 Australia

www.davidgillespie.org

ISBN 978-0-9874577-6-9

Design and layout: Charlotte Gelin Design
Photographs: iStock

Printed in Great Britain
by Amazon